The Plant-Based mix & match Cookbook

**A FLEXIBLE GUIDE TO BUILDING
NOURISH BOWLS, SALADS & HANDHELDS**

JEANNINE BILLUPS

Jeannine Billups
Kitchen is Love

kitchenislove.com
@kitchen.is.love

The Plant-Based Mix & Match Cookbook
A Flexible Guide to Building Nourish Bowls, Salads & Handhelds

First Edition

Softcover ISBN: 979-8-218-69633-7

Disclaimer: This book is for informational purposes only. While the recipes and suggestions provided are intended to promote a healthy plant-based lifestyle, they are not a substitute for professional medical advice or treatment. The author and publisher assume no responsibility for any errors, omissions, or outcomes resulting from the use of the recipes or recommendations in this book. The content is based on personal experience, research, and preferences and is intended for informational purposes only. Individual results may vary. Nutritional information has been provided by a registered dietitian; however, it should not be considered a substitute for professional medical or dietary advice. Always consult a qualified health-care provider before making significant changes to your diet or lifestyle.

Foreword by Dr. Kristi Artz

Cover & Book Design: Kristy Twellmann • umbrellasquared.com
Editor: Kelly Messier

Cover & Food Photography: Jeannine Billups
Initial concept & layout, illustrations, and lifestyle photography: Ted Billups

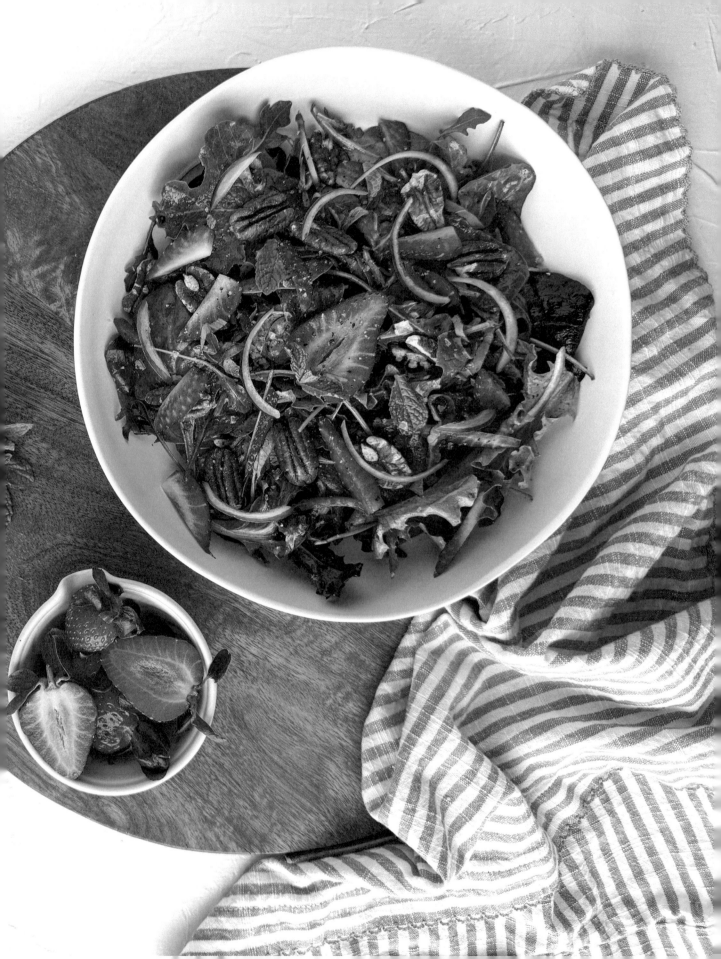

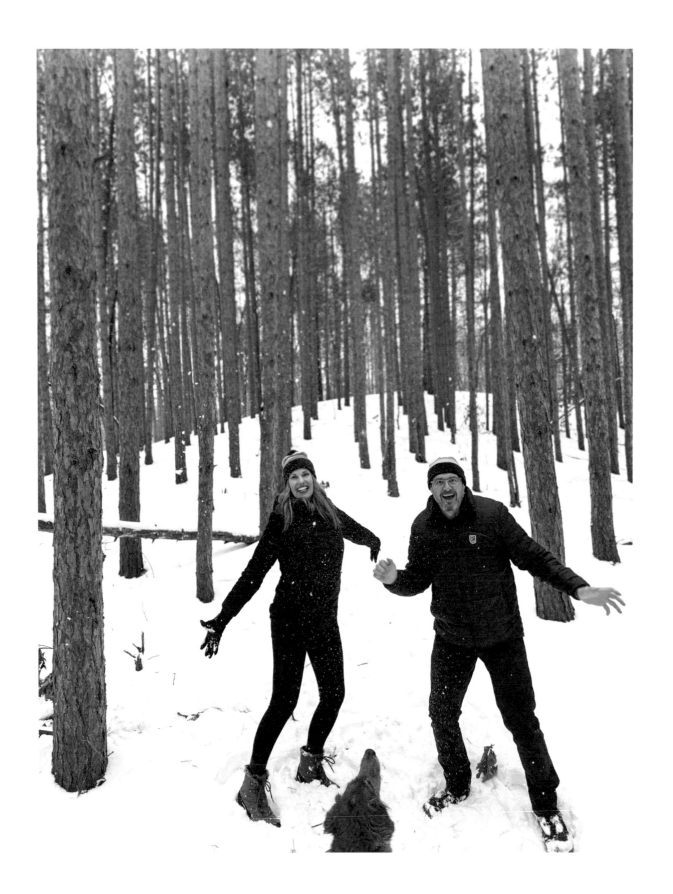

DEDICATED TO TED + LUNA

Thank you for filling our lives with love, laughter, trails, and bird seed!
My heart is full. ♡

Contents

Foreword

Eating plant-based has never been easier or more widely accepted. Over the past several years, interest in plant-based eating has grown, creating more options to explore delicious, whole plant foods in your daily nutrition plan. Reasons for moving toward this style of eating vary; some people cite personal health reasons, while others are inspired to align their dietary choices with the health of the planet. No matter how you have arrived at plant-based eating, you have come to the right place.

In 2019, the EAT-Lancet Commission published updated nutrition guidance to align economic, planetary, and population health goals.[1] This commission, composed of nutrition experts from around the world, named these recommendations the Planetary Health Diet. Notably, this diet highlights the substantial health benefits imparted to the individual and environment from eating a plant-rich diet. It allows for flexibility based on cultural preferences to ensure diets are delicious and sustainable. If you haven't read their brief, I encourage you to do so.

As a practicing physician with board certification in lifestyle and culinary medicine, I have daily conversations with patients about nutrition and health. Many share feelings of being overwhelmed by the constant onslaught of clickbait fad diets. They feel conflicted by perceived contradictions among nutrition experts. Most have great interest in achieving better health and would like to follow scientific evidence, yet are uncertain where to begin. The most straightforward advice I can provide is to add more whole plant foods in an enjoyable way. Do this early (in life) and often—your health will thrive while you'll be contributing to a healthier planet.

Whole plant foods include the incredible variety of vegetables, fruits, whole grains, legumes, nuts, seeds, herbs, and spices—all the components you will find artfully and thoughtfully presented by Jeannine, plant-based chef extraordinaire! Jeannine has supported the health of my family with weekly meal preparations of many (if not all) of the recipes you will find in this book. We particularly love the

Mushroom Walnut Taco Filling (page 103) with Cilantro Lime Crema (page 77) and request this as a frequent repeat. I recognize how incredibly fortunate we are to have the expertise of someone like Jeannine creating plant-based meals for our family. I share this with you to demonstrate just how much we value nutrition in our family. In my experience, when you get the nutrition right, most everything else tends to fall into place!

So whether you are a busy parent raising a family or an older adult trying to improve chronic health conditions, there is something here for everyone. I recommend you refer to the helpful guides on pantry and kitchen staples that Jeannine offers. Then jump right into preparing one of the simple and delicious plant-based bowls! There is immense flexibility in the way the material is presented here. You may even choose to add a little animal protein as a condiment to your plant-based bowl. This would still be in line with the Planetary Health Diet, giving you great confidence in your approach to health—for yourself, your family, and the planet.

In health,

Kristi Artz, MD
Board Certified Lifestyle and Emergency Medicine Physician;
Certified Culinary Medicine Specialist

Dr. Kristi Artz is a healthcare leader in Lifestyle Medicine, Culinary Medicine and Population Health. In her current role she leads a team of experts who research and provide evidence-based Integrative and Lifestyle Medicine services at a large academic health system in the Midwest. She frequently speaks on these topics at national conferences. You can find her on LinkedIn to learn more.

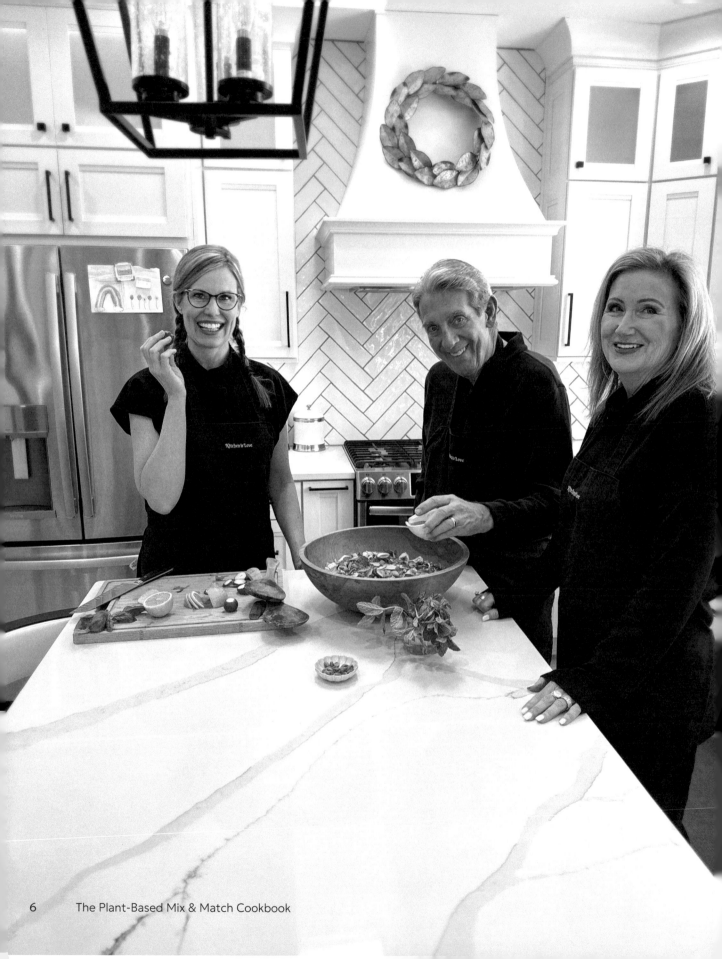

The Plant-Based Mix & Match Cookbook

Introduction

Welcome! I'm so happy you're here.
This cookbook is filled with tested and approved recipes designed for mix & match meals all week long. With versatile dressings, sauces, grains, and proteins, you'll save time, reduce waste, and keep meals fresh and exciting. Whether you're tossing a salad, building a nourish bowl, or wrapping up something flavorful, these recipes make healthy eating effortless and satisfying—all while being plant-based, refined sugar-free, and mostly gluten-free.

As a plant-based personal chef and culinary coach, I prepare weekly meals for clients and teach private in-home cooking classes. But it wasn't always this way. For over a decade, I struggled with health issues—including poor digestion, low energy, and heartburn—until I realized the direct connection between my diet and my overall well-being.

At the time, my busy sales job required daily travel, and I relied heavily on takeout and processed foods, rarely cooking at home. I knew I needed a change. I began incorporating more nutrient-dense whole foods while reducing processed foods, and the improvement was almost immediate. I felt a deep desire to share the love, so I pursued professional culinary training to help others achieve their health goals through simple, delicious plant-forward meals.

Customize, Experiment, and Enjoy
Food should fit your lifestyle, not the other way around! These recipes are fully customizable—swap ingredients, play with flavors, and adapt them to your family's needs. If you're cooking for mixed eaters, you can easily add a favorite animal protein while keeping the base plant-powered. This isn't a rule book—it's a flexible guide to help you nourish yourself, feel amazing, and love what's on your plate.

The Kitchen is Love Philosophy
The kitchen is the heart and soul of a home, a place where loved ones and guests migrate. We make daily decisions in the kitchen to either fuel our bodies with whole foods or consume processed foods that don't make us feel our best. Together, we can make healthier decisions—one step at a time—that show we care about ourselves, our loved ones, our community, and the planet.

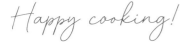

Happy cooking!

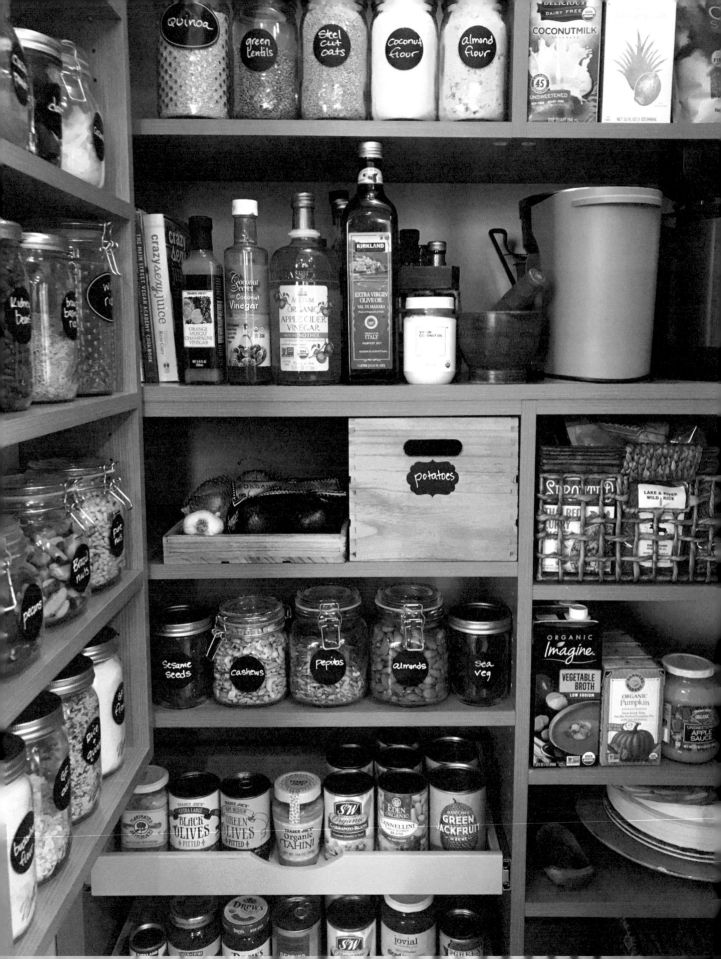

The Pantry

LET'S STOCK UP!

The Pantry List

A well-stocked kitchen and pantry offer numerous benefits, making cooking both efficient and enjoyable. **Here are some key advantages:**

Convenience: Saves time and reduces the need for frequent grocery trips.
Cost savings: Buying in bulk or during sales lowers food costs and reduces waste.
Healthy eating: Encourages nutritious meal choices with readily available whole foods.

Below, is a list of my most commonly used ingredients. While I have recommended specific brands that I prefer, feel free to use similar ingredients that are easily accessible to you. Whenever possible, avoid unnecessary additives like artificial colors, preservatives, added sodium, and refined sugars.

REFRIGERATOR

- ○ Nondairy yogurt (plain, unsweetened cashew, or coconut)
- ○ Organic Miso Master White Mellow Miso (or chickpea miso)
- ○ Organic shelled edamame
- ○ Organic tempeh
- ○ Organic tofu (firm, extra-firm, and super-firm)

PANTRY

- ○ Arrowroot starch (or non-GMO cornstarch)
- ○ Bread (sourdough, whole wheat, whole-grain pita, naan)
- ○ Canned beans (black, cannellini, red kidney)
- ○ Canned chickpeas
- ○ Canned lentils (brown or green)
- ○ Dried fruit, unsweetened (cherries, cranberries, dates)
- ○ Dry whole grains (brown rice, farro, quinoa)
- ○ Marinara sauce
- ○ Noodles (brown rice, chickpea, lentil, quinoa, soba, whole wheat)
- ○ Raw nuts and seeds (cashews, walnuts, pecans, almonds, hemp hearts, flaxseed meal)
- ○ Ready-to-heat whole grains (brown rice, quinoa)
- ○ Toasted nuts and seeds (sliced almonds, peanuts, sesame seeds)
- ○ Vegetable broth or bouillon, low-sodium
- ○ Mangos
- ○ Mushrooms (cremini, white button)
- ○ Onions
- ○ Pineapple
- ○ Potatoes
- ○ Radishes
- ○ Shallots
- ○ Sweet potatoes
- ○ Tomatoes

CONDIMENTS

- ◯ Dijon mustard
- ◯ Frank's Original RedHot Cayenne Pepper Sauce
- ◯ Kalamata olives, pitted
- ◯ Natural nut and seed butter (peanut, almond, cashew, sunflower)
- ◯ Pure maple syrup
- ◯ San-J Organic Reduced Sodium Tamari (25% less sodium)
- ◯ San-J Organic Tamari Lite (50% less sodium)
- ◯ Sriracha
- ◯ Tahini
- ◯ Vegan mayonnaise

OILS + VINEGARS

- ◯ Aged balsamic vinegar
- ◯ Balsamic glaze
- ◯ Extra-virgin olive oil
- ◯ Raw apple cider vinegar
- ◯ Red wine vinegar
- ◯ Rice vinegar
- ◯ Toasted sesame oil
- ◯ White wine vinegar

PRODUCE

- ◯ Apples
- ◯ Asparagus
- ◯ Bell peppers (red, orange, yellow)
- ◯ Broccoli
- ◯ Brussels sprouts
- ◯ Cabbage (red, green, Napa)
- ◯ Carrots
- ◯ Celery
- ◯ Citrus fruit (limes, lemons, navel oranges, mandarin oranges)
- ◯ Cucumbers
- ◯ Garlic cloves
- ◯ Ginger, raw
- ◯ Herbs (fresh cilantro, parsley, basil, mint, dill)
- ◯ Jalapeño
- ◯ Kale, curly

SPICES

- ◯ Crushed red pepper flakes
- ◯ Curry powder
- ◯ Dried dill
- ◯ Dried oregano
- ◯ Dried thyme
- ◯ Freshly ground black pepper
- ◯ Garlic powder
- ◯ Ground cayenne pepper
- ◯ Ground cumin
- ◯ Ground sumac
- ◯ Ground turmeric
- ◯ Nutritional yeast
- ◯ Onion powder
- ◯ Paprika (sweet and smoked)
- ◯ Salt (kosher, sea salt)

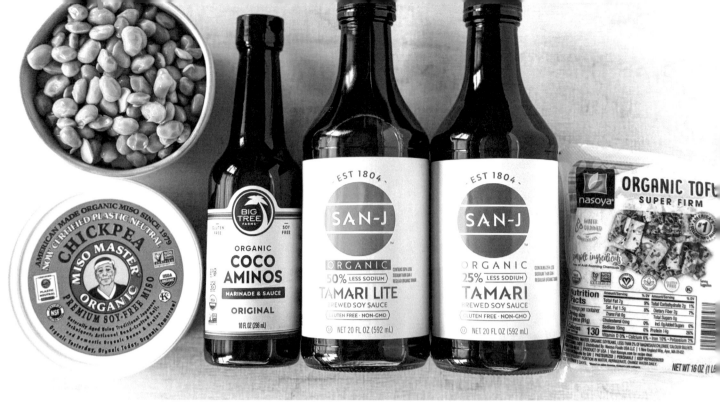

Soy Products

Choose organic and/or non-GMO soy products whenever possible as soy is commonly genetically modified in the U.S. This includes tofu, tempeh, edamame, soy sauce, tamari, and miso paste.

Soy Sauce vs. Tamari vs. Coconut Aminos
All three sauces add a salty and umami depth of flavor to recipes and can be used interchangeably. Ingredients and sodium levels vary in each product.

Soy sauce: Traditionally made from fermented soybeans, wheat, water, and salt. Contains soy and gluten. Choose versions with 50% less sodium whenever possible.

Tamari: Typically made from fermented soybeans and little or no wheat. Gluten-free varieties available. Has a slightly thicker texture and a more mellow flavor compared with soy sauce. Choose Tamari Lite (50% less sodium) whenever possible.

Coconut aminos: Made from fermented sap of coconut palm and sea salt. Naturally gluten-free and soy-free, making it a good option for those avoiding soy or gluten. Has a slightly sweeter and milder flavor compared with soy sauce and tamari. Typically lower in sodium compared with soy sauce and tamari, depending on the brand.

Kitchen Tool List

Here are my most-used kitchen tools. While not all are essential, they'll save you time and effort! If you're missing any, check local dollar stores or resale shops; I've found some great gems over the years.

- ◯ 1 large nonstick skillet with lid
- ◯ 1 medium saucepan with lid
- ◯ 1-cup and 2-cup glass measuring cups
- ◯ 1-cup storage containers with airtight lids
- ◯ 2 large rimmed baking sheets
- ◯ 4 oz condiment containers with airtight lids
- ◯ 8-cup storage containers with airtight lids
- ◯ 12-cup food processor*
- ◯ Air fryer (optional)
- ◯ Chef's knife
- ◯ Citrus press
- ◯ Cutting boards

- ◯ Garlic press
- ◯ High-speed blender*
- ◯ Measuring spoons
- ◯ Microplane
- ◯ Mixing bowl set
- ◯ Parchment paper
- ◯ Paring knife (serrated)
- ◯ Pint-size canning jars with lids (wide mouth)
- ◯ Silicone spatula
- ◯ Slotted spoon
- ◯ Spatula
- ◯ Whisk

*Note:

A high-speed blender creates smooth and creamy sauces, dressings, and smoothies. A food processor is used to mince mushrooms and walnuts. Alternatively, you can chop these ingredients by hand.

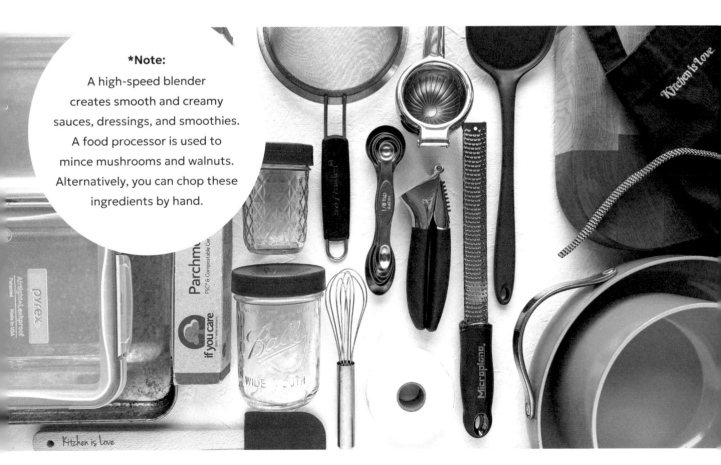

Tips Before We Get Started

Batch Cooking

When time is tight, ready-to-heat grains and canned beans are lifesavers.
For those who prefer cooking from scratch, batch cooking is your best friend!

1. Dedicate one day each month to prepare large quantities of staples like black beans and brown rice.
2. After cooking, let them cool, then portion into reusable freezer bags. These can be frozen for up to 3 months.
3. Thaw what you need in the fridge for quick additions to salads, nourish bowls, handhelds, soup, & stews.

Shopping

Save time, money, and reduce food waste with these tips:

Shop at home: Check your fridge and pantry first to find items that need to be used or might be going bad.

Use prepped foods: Buy items like toasted nuts, canned beans, shredded carrots, cabbage slaw, and frozen produce to save prep time.

Buy in bulk: Get great deals on staples like grains, beans, frozen produce, nut butters, nondairy milks, and tofu at warehouse clubs.

Purchase seasonal produce: Shop at farmers markets for fresh in-season fruits and vegetables. They taste better, last longer, and support your local community.

Eating the Rainbow

Incorporating these fiber-filled colorful plant foods into your meals ensures a wide range of nutrients and health benefits! Some examples include:

- Red (tomatoes, red peppers, strawberries, beets)
- Orange (carrots, sweet potatoes, butternut squash, oranges)
- Yellow (pineapple, corn, yellow bell peppers, lemons)
- Green (spinach, kale, broccoli, avocados)
- Blue/Purple (blueberries, eggplant, cabbage, blackberries)
- White/Brown (cauliflower, mushrooms, garlic, onions)

A few more things to keep in mind ...

Start small: If you're new to meal prep, begin by prepping a small amount of food. Gradually increase the amount as you become more comfortable.

Efficiency grows: The more you make a recipe, the faster and more efficient you'll become. Keep a list of your favorites and rotate them monthly.

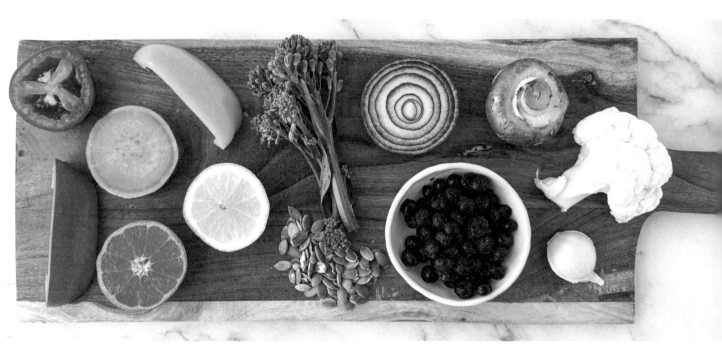

*You've got this.
I believe in you!*

Let's
CREATE!

In this chapter, we will explore the concept of weekly meal planning and mix & match meal creation. I share a sample of my weekly meal planning and prep process, and then tie it all together with flexible mix & match meal charts so that you can create your own customized salads, nourish bowls, and handhelds. Lastly, I will share examples of our favorite meals to help fill you with inspiration!

- Weekly Meal Planning + Prep
- How to Build Mix & Match Meals
- Meal Inspiration

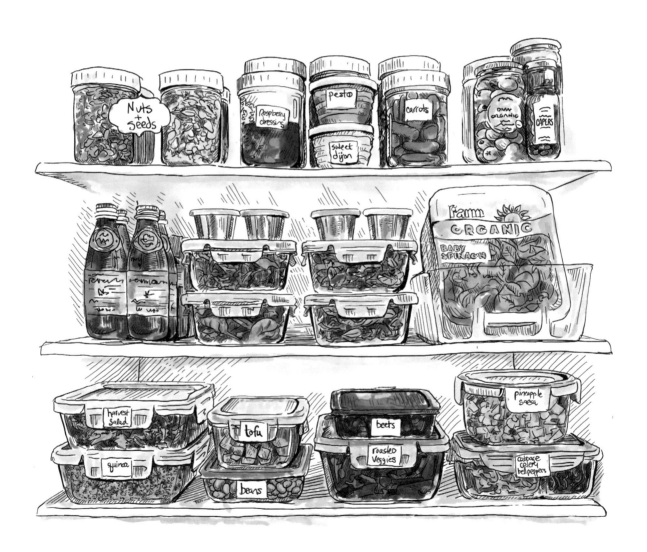

Weekly Meal Planning + Prep

Most people don't want to eat the same meal more than twice a week, but they still want simplicity. My solution is prepping individual meal components. Think Chipotle! A batch of rice, beans, roasted and raw veggies, and flavorful sauces. These ingredients can be mixed and matched throughout the week to create a variety of meals, in as little as five minutes each! **Almost every week, usually on a Sunday, I spend one to two hours preparing the components. Here is my process:**

1. Create a Meal Plan

Choose one or more flavors you are craving:
- ○ American
- ○ Mediterranean
- ○ Latin
- ○ Asian

Choose two or more types of meals you are craving:
- ○ Nourish bowls
- ○ Salads
- ○ Tacos
- ○ Wraps

Shop your kitchen:
- Check your fridge and pantry first to find items that you already have on hand or that might be going bad.
- Write these ingredients on a shopping list.

Select your recipes:
- Based on your cravings and available ingredients, choose your components and recipes. Aim for one batch each of rice, legumes, and roasted and raw veggies, as well as flavorful sauces.
- Create a shopping list.
- Check off items you already have.

2. Go Shopping

- ○ Go shopping at your local grocery store and farmers market or use a grocery delivery service. *(can be done 1 or 2 days in advance)*

3. Set Up Your Kitchen

1. Empty the dishwasher for easy cleanup.
2. Clear and clean counters.
3. Gather all ingredients and tools.
4. Reuse tools and do quick washes between recipes to minimize dishes.

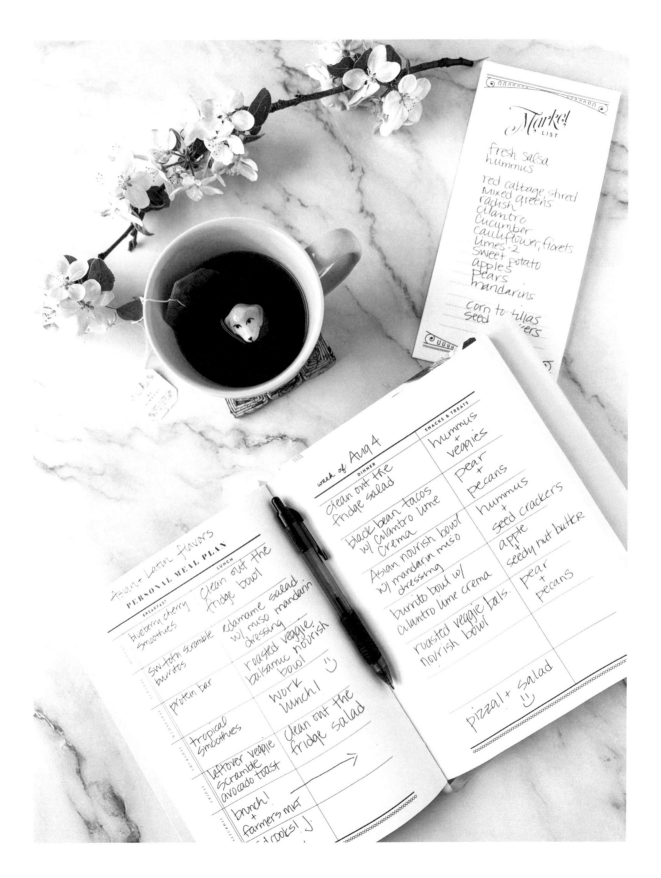

Market List

fresh salsa
hummus

red cabbage shred
Mixed greens
radish
cilantro
cucumber
cauliflower florets
limes - 2
sweet potato
apples
pears
mandarins

corn tortillas
seed ~~crackers~~

Asian + Latin Flavors

PERSONAL MEAL PLAN

	BREAKFAST	LUNCH
	Blueberry cherry smoothies	Clean out the fridge bowl
	Sw tofu scramble burritos	edamame salad w/ miso mandarin dressing
	protein bar	roasted veggie balsamic nourish bowl
	tropical smoothies	Work lunch! ☺
	Leftover veggie scramble avocado toast	Clean out the fridge salad →
	brunch! + farmers mkt	

week of Aug 4

DINNER	SNACKS & TREATS
clean out the fridge salad	hummus + veggies
black bean tacos w/ cilantro lime crema	pear + pecans
Asian nourish bowl w/ mandarin miso dressing	hummus + seed crackers
burrito bowl w/ cilantro lime crema	apple + seedy nut butter
roasted veggie balls nourish bowl	pear + pecans
pizza! + salad ☺	

4. Make The Food

Review the recipes:
Read the entire recipe from beginning to end to become familiar with the preparation/cooking process and timing.

Make the food:
Start by making the individual recipe components that take the longest to cook and cool. For example, cook the rice and roast the vegetables first. In the meantime, prep the raw veggies, heat the beans and edamame, and make the sauce and dressing.

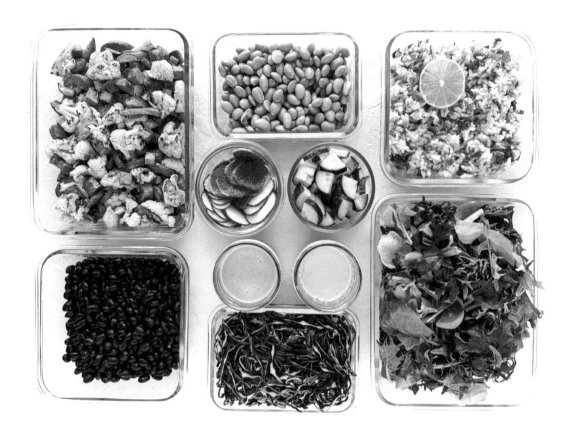

Top row (L to R):
- Roasted cauliflower, sweet potatoes, and carrots (page 87)
- Sesame Tamari Edamame (page 29)
- Cilantro Lime Rice (page 147)

Middle row (L to R):
- Sliced radishes
- Diced cucumbers
- Cilantro Lime Crema (page 77)
- Mandarin Miso Dressing (page 63)

Bottom row (L to R):
- Easy Beans (page 111)
- Sliced red cabbage
- Prewashed salad greens

5. Store The Food

1. Allow the food to cool.
2. Store each component in individual storage containers.
3. Label each container.

6. Create Your Mix & Match Meals

1. Create a flexible menu and stick it on the fridge.
2. Mix and match components during the week, reheating with the microwave, stovetop, or enjoy cold depending on the meal.

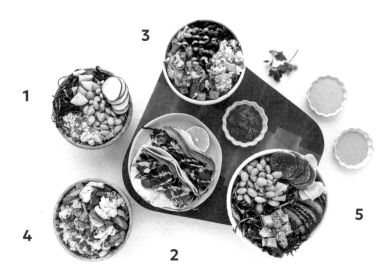

1. **Edamame Salad with Mandarin Miso Dressing:** salad greens + red cabbage + radish + cucumber + edamame + Mandarin Miso Dressing
2. **Black Bean Tacos with Cilantro Lime Crema:** Easy Black Beans + red cabbage + tomatoes + avocado + salsa
3. **Burrito Bowl with Cilantro Lime Crema:** Cilantro Lime Rice + roasted veggies + Easy Black Beans + Cilantro Lime Crema
4. **Roasted Veggie Balsamic Nourish Bowl:** Cilantro Lime Rice + roasted veggies + extra-virgin olive oil & balsamic vinegar drizzle + salt & pepper
5. **Asian Nourish Bowl with Mandarin Miso Dressing:** Cilantro Lime Rice + red cabbage + cucumber + radish + edamame + Mandarin Miso Dressing

How to Build Mix & Match Meals

Making tasty, healthy salads, nourish bowls, and handhelds is a breeze with this simple formula! Just pick from each category below to create a meal that will tickle your tastebuds. If your favorite ingredient isn't listed, go ahead and add it in!

STEP 1

BASE

Select one type of meal: a salad, nourish bowl, or handheld.

Salad
(1 ½ packed cups of one or more)
- Arugula
- Baby spinach
- Cabbage
- Kale
- Mixed greens
- Romaine lettuce

Nourish Bowl
(½–¾ cup of one or more)
- Brown rice
- Farro
- Quinoa
- Sweet potatoes
- Whole-grain or legume pasta

Handheld
(1 or 2 pieces)
- Sourdough bread
- Whole-grain tortilla
- Whole-grain wrap
- Whole wheat pita

STEP 2

PROTEIN

Select ½ cup of one or more and layer on top of the BASE.

- Black, red kidney, cannellini, and/or refried beans
- Chickpeas
- Edamame
- Lentils
- Quinoa
- Tofu
- Tempeh

STEP 3

ROASTED VEGGIES

Select ½ to 2 cups of a variety of roasted vegetables and layer on top of the PROTEIN. Refer to the roasting chart (page 87) for the cooking method.

- Asparagus
- Beets
- Bell peppers
- Broccoli
- Brussels sprouts
- Butternut squash
- Cauliflower
- Mushrooms
- Onions
- Potatoes
- Sweet potatoes
- Tomatoes
- Zucchini

STEP 4

RAW VEGGIES
Select ½ cup of a variety of rainbow-colored vegetables and layer on top of the ROASTED VEGGIES.

- Bell peppers
- Cabbage
- Carrots
- Celery
- Corn
- Cucumbers
- Radishes
- Tomatoes

STEP 5

FLAVOR
Select 2 tablespoons of one or more and layer on top of the RAW VEGGIES.

- Aged balsamic vinegar
- Extra-virgin olive oil and vinegar
- Homemade dressing or sauce (refer to "Flavor" chapter for recipes)

STEP 6

TOPPERS
Select 2 tablespoons or more and layer on top of the FLAVOR.

- Avocado
- Fermented vegetables
- Fresh fruit (apples, berries, grapes, mandarin oranges)
- Fresh herbs
- Hummus
- Microgreens
- Salsa
- Olives
- Onions
- Toasted nuts or seeds
- Tomatoes
- Unsweetened dried fruit (cherries, cranberries, dates, raisins)

MEAL
Inspirations

FOR THOSE OF US THAT NEED
A LITTLE INSPIRATION, HERE ARE SOME
EXAMPLES OF OUR FAVORITE MEALS.

Salad Inspirations

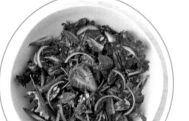

Strawberry Pecan Salad
- Spring mix
- Toasted pecans
- Red onion
- Strawberries
- Aged balsamic vinegar and olive oil
- Fresh mint and basil leaves

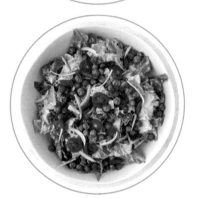

Caesar Salad
- Romaine lettuce
- Roasted Chickpeas (page 109)
- Red onion
- Kalamata olives
- Tomatoes
- Cashew Caesar Dressing (page 45)

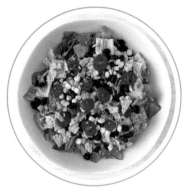

Southwest Salad
- Romaine lettuce
- Black beans
- Corn kernels
- Red onion
- Tomatoes
- Crushed tortilla chips
- Creamy Cilantro Dressing (page 73)

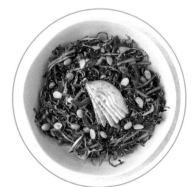

Edamame Crunch Salad
- Cabbage Slaw
- Shelled edamame
- Matchstick carrots
- Red bell pepper
- Avocado
- Green onions
- Toasted almonds and sesame seeds
- Orange Sesame Sauce (page 65)

Nourish Bowl Inspirations

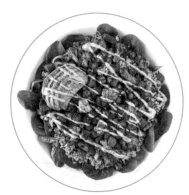

Roasted Harvest Bowl

- Baby spinach
- Quinoa
- Roasted Chickpeas (page 109)
- Roasted sweet potatoes + cauliflower (page 87)
- Avocado
- Sweet Dijon Dressing (page 33)

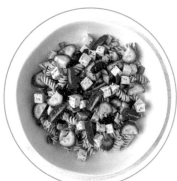

Greek Pasta Salad

- Whole-grain pasta
- Mediterranean Tofu Feta (page 123)
- Green bell pepper
- Cucumber
- Tomatoes
- Kalamata olives
- Fresh herbs
- Greek Vinaigrette (page 47)

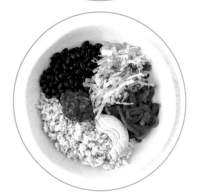

Burrito Bowl

- Brown rice
- Easy Beans (page 107)
- Sautéed Bell Peppers (page 99)
- Lettuce
- Salsa
- Avocado

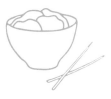

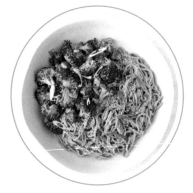

Peanut Soba Bowl

- Soba noodles
- Sautéed Broccoli (page 97)
- Peanut Ginger Sauce (page 67)
- Toasted sesame seeds
- Green onions

Handheld Inspirations

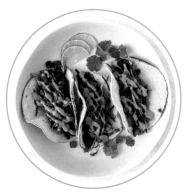

Chili Lime Bean Tacos
- Corn tortillas
- Easy Beans (page 107)
- Red cabbage
- Tomatoes
- Cilantro Lime Crema (page 77)

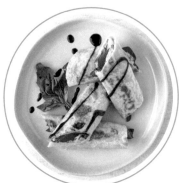

Basil Hummus Wraps
- Whole-grain wraps
- Hummus
- Lettuce
- Tomatoes
- Balsamic glaze
- Fresh basil

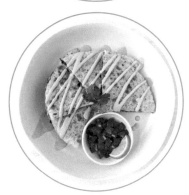

Fajita Quesadillas
- Whole wheat tortillas
- Refried beans, vegetarian
- Sautéed Bell Peppers (page 99)
- Tomatoes
- Cashew Queso (page 75)

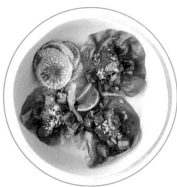

Asian Lettuce Wraps
- Butterhead lettuce cups
- Sweet Sriracha Tofu Cubes (page 121)
- Chopped peanuts
- Fresh cilantro leaves
- Radish

FLAVOR

Dressings, Sauces, and Salsas

When you make your own sauces and dressings, you can amplify flavor while reducing the adverse effects of highly processed oils, refined sugars, and excess sodium commonly found in store-bought products.

Incorporate naturally anti-inflammatory herbs and spices like turmeric, garlic, cilantro, and ginger, and pair them with heart-healthy monounsaturated and polyunsaturated fats from nuts, seeds, olives, and avocados—you'll feel the difference. What a great reason to season!

American-Inspired
- Creamy Basil Dressing
- Sweet Dijon Dressing
- Buffalo Sauce
- Maple Balsamic Dressing
- Raspberry Balsamic Dressing
- Apple Tahini Dressing
- Cashew Cream

Mediterranean-Inspired
- Cashew Caesar Dressing
- Greek Vinaigrette
- Creamy Greek Dressing
- Balsamic Walnut Dressing
- Alfredo Sauce
- Dill Sauce
- Citrus Tahini Sauce
- Basil Spinach Pesto
- Tzatziki Sauce

Asian-Inspired
- Mandarin Miso Dressing
- Orange Sesame Sauce
- Peanut Ginger Sauce
- Sesame Tahini Dressing
- Ginger Turmeric Vinaigrette

Latin-Inspired
- Creamy Cilantro Dressing
- Cashew Queso
- Cilantro Lime Crema

Salsas
- Pineapple Salsa
- Pico de Gallo
- Mango Salsa

Tips:

For all recipes that require a high-speed blender, using the smaller cup will allow you to remove most of the blended ingredients with ease and reduce waste. If you're using the larger blender cup, you may want to double the ingredient amounts in order to create a smooth and creamy consistency.

Many nut- and seed-based recipes may thicken after refrigeration. Give them a good whisk to soften— if they're still too thick, whisk in a teaspoon of cold water until desired consistency is reached.

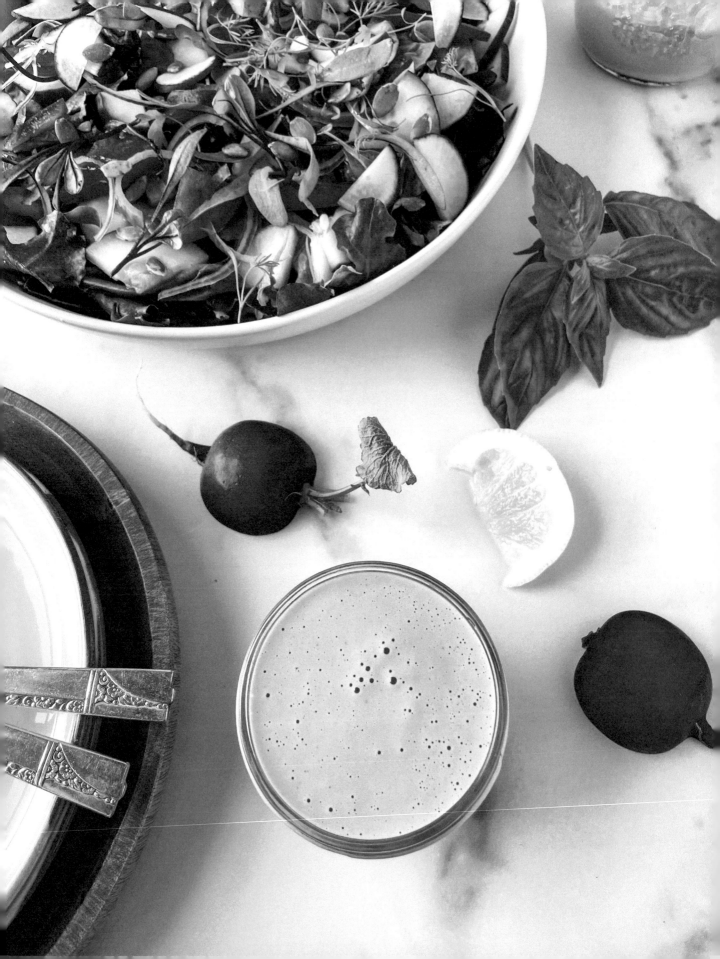

Creamy Basil Dressing

Makes about 4 servings

This ranch-like dressing is bursting with fresh basil and gets its creaminess from cashews. Drizzle it over crisp salads, toss it into chilled pasta salads, or use it as a creamy dip for fresh veggies.

INGREDIENTS

- ½ cup raw cashews, *see note**
- ½ cup packed fresh basil leaves
- ⅓ cup water
- ½ tablespoon fresh lemon juice
- 1 medium garlic clove, chopped
- 1 teaspoon white wine vinegar
- ½ teaspoon salt

METHOD

1. Combine all the ingredients in a high-speed blender and blend until smooth and creamy.
2. Chill for at least 30 minutes before serving.
3. Refrigerate leftovers in an airtight container for up to four days.

*Note:
If you don't have a high-speed blender, soak the cashews in hot water for 15 minutes prior to blending. Discard soaking water and proceed as directed.

NUTRITIONAL INFORMATION (PER SERVING)

Calories 92.1, Carbohydrate 5.4 g, Fiber 0.6 g, Total Sugars 1 g, Added Sugars 0g, Fat 7.2 g, Saturated Fat 1.3 g, Protein 3.1 g, Sodium 297.7 mg, Iron 1.2 mg

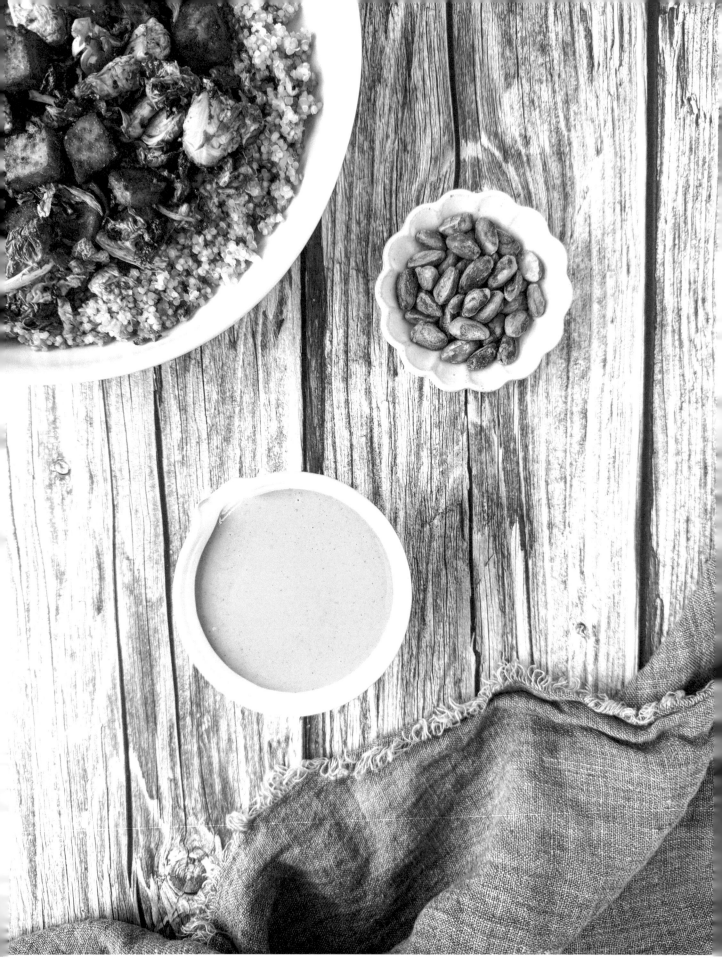

Sweet Dijon Dressing

Makes about 4 servings

This is an amplified version of honey mustard dressing, which is a client favorite! It pairs well with bitter veggies like brussels sprouts and dark leafy greens. Sweet Dijon Dressing also makes an irresistible dipping sauce for sweet potato fries.

INGREDIENTS

- 3 tablespoons tahini
- 3 tablespoons Dijon mustard
- 3 tablespoons pure maple syrup
- 1 tablespoon raw apple cider vinegar
- 1 tablespoon fresh lemon juice

METHOD

1. In a small bowl, combine the tahini, Dijon, maple syrup, vinegar, and lemon juice. Whisk together until super smooth and creamy. If the sauce is too thick, add a tablespoon of ice-cold water at a time until you reach a pourable consistency. This will vary depending on the thickness of your tahini.

2. Serve cold or at room temperature.

3. Refrigerate in an airtight container for up to 7 days.

NUTRITIONAL INFORMATION (PER SERVING)

Per serving: Calories 117.6, Carbohydrate 13.3 g, Fiber 1.4 g, Total Sugars 9.4 g, Added Sugars 8.9 g, Fat 6.7 g, Saturated Fat 0.9 g, Protein 2.4 g, Sodium 284.4 mg, Iron 1.3 mg

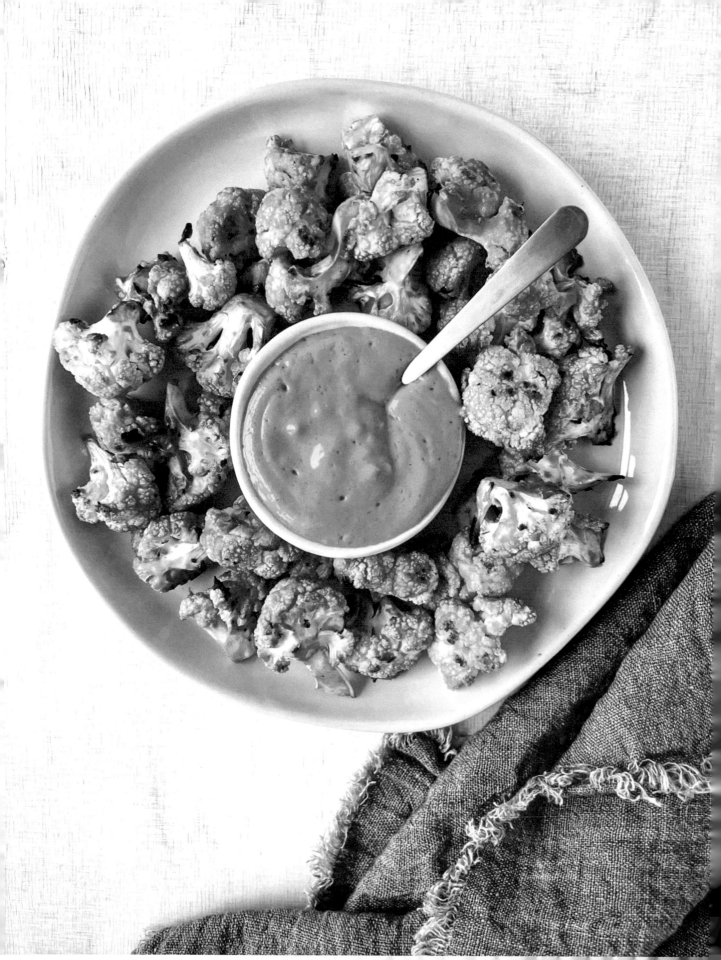

Buffalo Sauce

Makes about 6 servings

This often-requested sauce pairs well with crumbled tofu or tempeh wrapped in a whole-grain tortilla topped with crunchy celery and a dollop of creamy Dill Sauce (page 55).

INGREDIENTS

- ⅓ cup Frank's RedHot Original Cayenne Pepper Sauce
- ⅓ cup water
- 3 tablespoons raw cashews, *see note**
- 2 tablespoons Tamari Lite
- ¾ tablespoon pure maple syrup
- 2 teaspoons white wine vinegar
- 1 teaspoon garlic powder

METHOD

1. Put all the ingredients in a high-speed blender and blend until smooth.
2. Serve warm or at room temperature.
3. Refrigerate leftovers in an airtight container for up to 7 days.

*Note:
If you don't have
a high-speed blender,
soak the cashews in hot water
for 15 minutes prior to blending.
Discard soaking water and proceed
as directed.

If you have a tree-nut allergy,
omit the cashews and add
3 tablespoons of
hemp hearts

NUTRITIONAL INFORMATION (PER SERVING)

Per serving: Calories 35.4, Carbohydrate 3.8 g, Fiber 0.2 g, Total Sugars 1.9 g, Added Sugars 1.5 g, Fat 1.8 g, Saturated Fat 0.3 g, Protein 1.2 g, Sodium 671.6 mg, Iron 0.7 mg

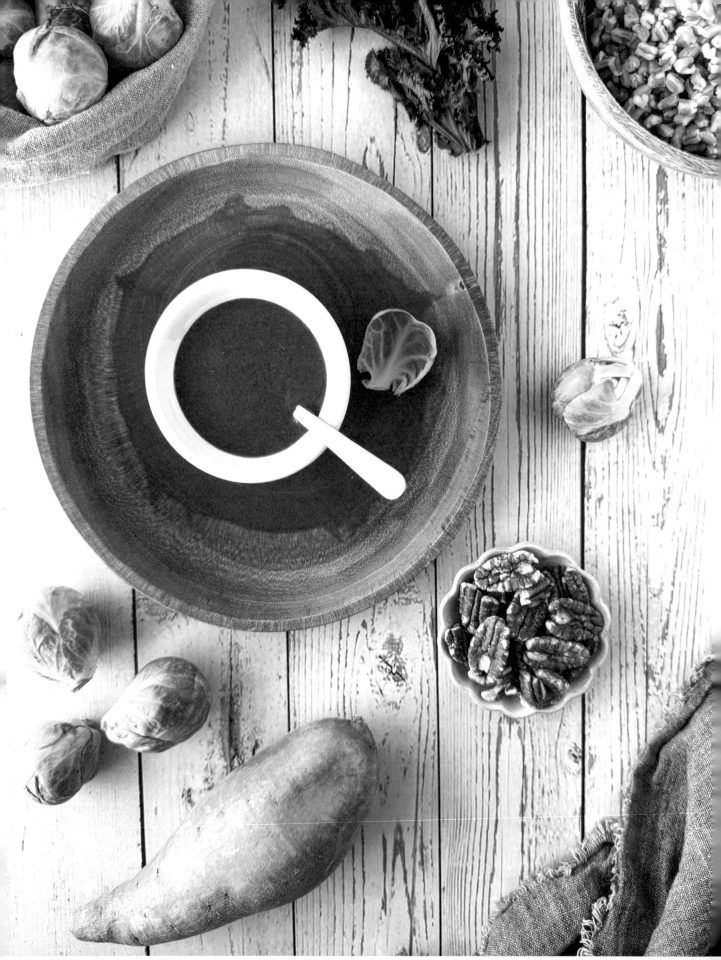

Maple Balsamic Dressing

Makes about 4 servings

This rich and creamy oil-free dressing is made with aged balsamic vinegar and tahini. Drizzle it over roasted squash and Brussels sprouts, served on a bed of farro or fresh salad greens topped with crisp apples and toasted pecans.

INGREDIENTS

- 2 tablespoons tahini
- 2 tablespoons ice-cold water
- 2 tablespoons aged balsamic vinegar
- 1 tablespoon pure maple syrup
- ¼ teaspoon ground cinnamon
- ¼ teaspoon dried thyme, finely chopped

METHOD

1. Combine the tahini and water in a small bowl and whisk together until super smooth and creamy. Add the remaining ingredients and whisk until well combined. If the sauce is too thick, add a teaspoon of ice-cold water at a time until you reach a pourable consistency. This will vary depending on the thickness of your tahini.
2. Serve cold or at room temperature.
3. Refrigerate leftovers in an airtight container for up to 7 days.

NUTRITIONAL INFORMATION (PER SERVING)

Per serving: Calories 73, Carbohydrate 8.6 g, Fiber 0.8 g, Total Sugars 6.1 g, Added Sugars 3 g, Fat 4 g, Saturated Fat 0.6, Protein 1.3 g, Sodium 12.2 mg, Iron 0.9 mg

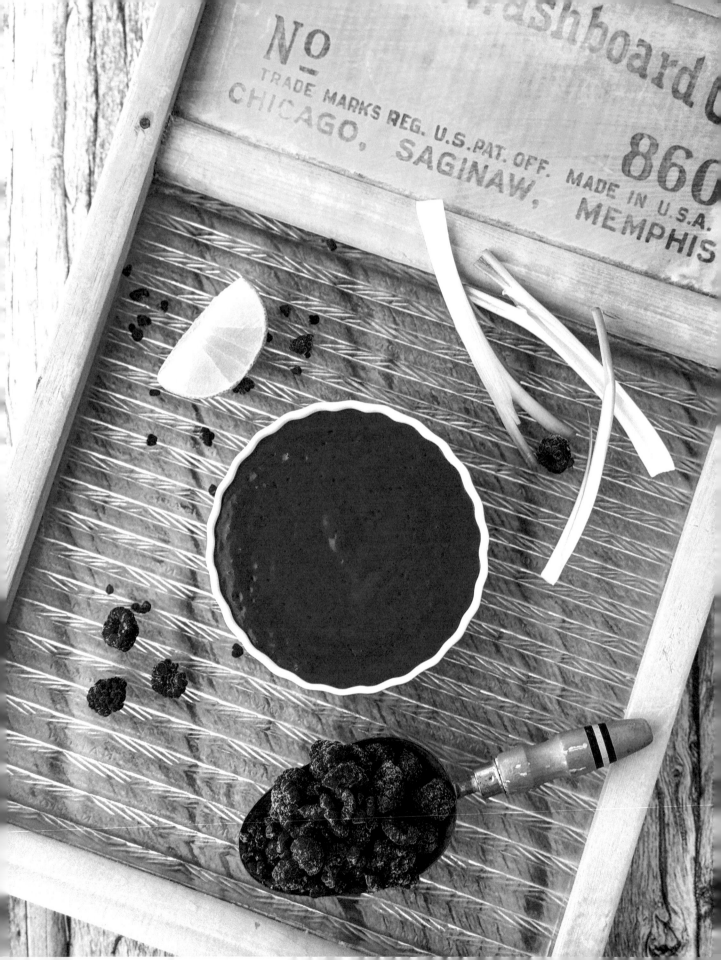

Raspberry Balsamic Dressing

Makes about 5 servings

Raspberries are blended with balsamic vinegar, aromatics, citrus juice, and maple syrup. It pairs perfectly with a summer berry salad of mixed greens, fresh strawberries and blueberries, red onion, and toasted nuts.

INGREDIENTS

- 1 cup raspberries, fresh or frozen
- ¼ cup water, more as needed
- 3 tablespoons extra-virgin olive oil
- 3 tablespoons aged balsamic vinegar
- 1 tablespoon fresh lime, lemon, or orange juice
- 1-inch piece green onion, white and light green parts only, chopped
- 1 tablespoon pure maple syrup
- ¼ teaspoon salt

METHOD

1. Put all the ingredients in a high-speed blender and blend until smooth and creamy. Add additional water as needed to reach a pourable consistency.
2. Chill for at least 30 minutes before serving.
3. Refrigerate in an airtight container for up to 3 days. Shake well before serving.
4. The dressing will thicken once refrigerated. Add a teaspoon of cold water until you reach desired consistency.

NUTRITIONAL INFORMATION (PER SERVING)

Per serving: Calories 113.5, Carbohydrate 10.1 g, Fiber 1.6 g, Total Sugars 7.1 g, Added Sugars 2.4 g, Fat 8.3 g, Saturated Fat 1.1 g, Protein 0.3 g, Sodium 122.4 mg, Iron 0.4 mg

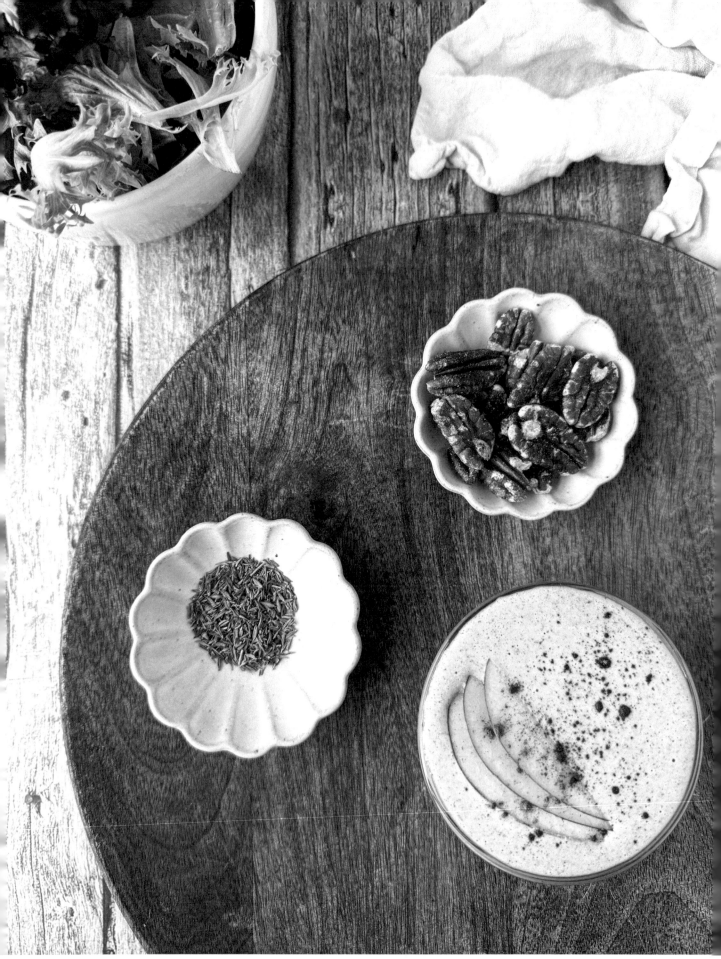

Apple Tahini Dressing

Makes about 6 servings

This tahini-based dressing, blended with apple, cinnamon, and a touch of maple syrup, is one of our favorite cold-weather dressings. It pairs beautifully with roasted squash, beets, dark leafy greens, dried cranberries, and toasted nuts.

INGREDIENTS

- ¼ cup tahini
- ¼ cup ice-cold water
- 1 medium red apple, cored and chopped into bite-size pieces
- 1 tablespoon raw apple cider vinegar
- 1 tablespoon pure maple syrup
- 1 medium garlic clove
- ½ teaspoon dried thyme
- ½ teaspoon ground cinnamon
- ¼ teaspoon salt

METHOD

1. Put all the ingredients in a high-speed blender and blend until smooth and creamy.
2. Chill for at least 30 minutes before serving.
3. Refrigerate leftovers in an airtight container for up to 5 days.
4. The dressing will thicken once refrigerated. Add a teaspoon of cold water until you reach desired consistency.

NUTRITIONAL INFORMATION (PER SERVING)

Per serving: Calories 85.3, Carbohydrate 8.9 g, Fiber 1.8 g, Total Sugars 5.3 g, Added Sugars 2 g, Fat 5.4 g, Saturated Fat 0.8 g, Protein 1.8 g, Sodium 111 mg, Iron 1.1 mg

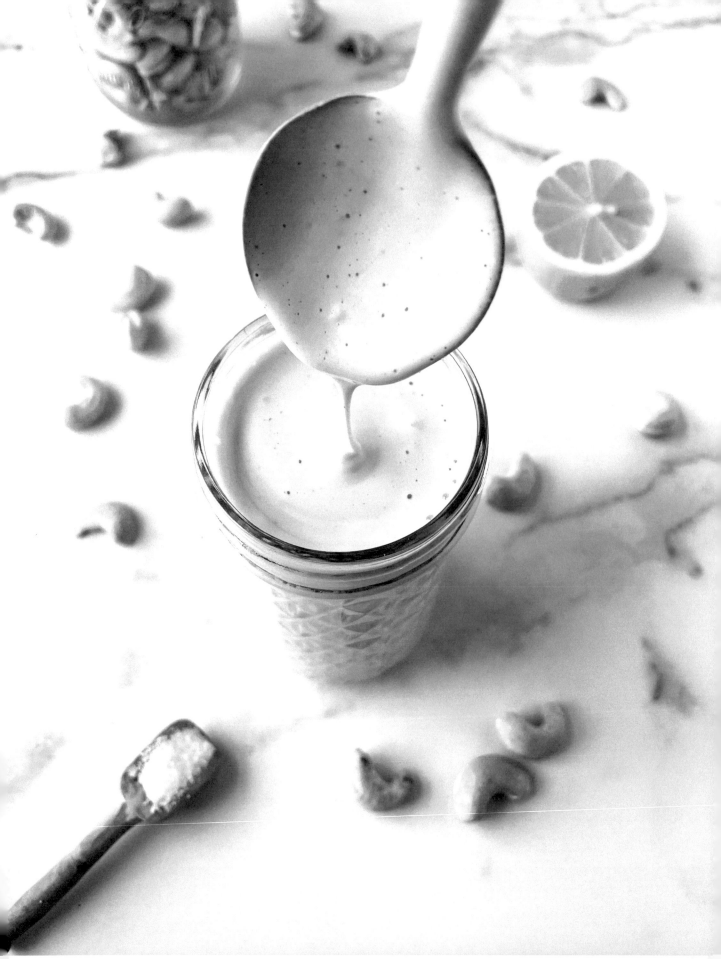

Cashew Cream

Makes about 8 servings

A versatile dairy-free alternative to regular cream that adds richness to savory dishes. Add to creamy soups, curries, pasta, and casseroles. Use Cashew Cream as the base of a creamy sauce or dressing, or in place of vegan mayonnaise.

INGREDIENTS

- 1 cup raw cashews, *see note**
- ¾ cup water
- 1 tablespoon fresh lemon juice
- ½ teaspoon salt

METHOD

1. Put all the ingredients in a high-speed blender. Blend together until you reach a smooth and creamy consistency, scraping sides as needed.
2. Refrigerate leftovers in an airtight container for up to a week.

*Note:
If you don't have a high-speed blender, soak the cashews in hot water for 15 minutes prior to blending. Discard soaking water and proceed as directed.

NUTRITIONAL INFORMATION (PER SERVING)

Per serving: Calories 90.3, Carbohydrate 5 g, Fiber 0.5 g, Total Sugars 1 g, Added Sugars 0 g, Fat 7.1 g, Saturated Fat 1.3 g, Protein 3 g, Sodium 150.2 mg, Iron 1.1 mg

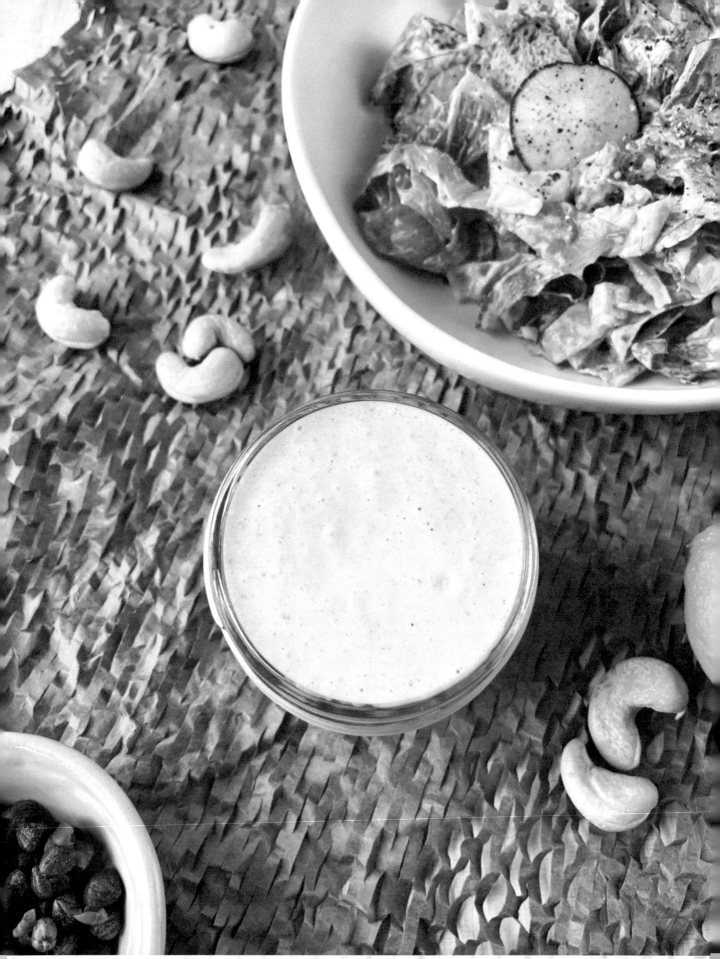

Cashew Caesar Dressing

Makes about 4 servings

This is one of my most requested dressings, and a recipe I whip up every two weeks for my family! The cashew-based dressing pairs well with crispy romaine, kale, and roasted chickpeas, whether enjoyed as a vibrant salad or tucked into a whole-grain wrap.

INGREDIENTS

- ½ cup raw cashews, *see note**
- ½ cup water
- 2 tablespoons lemon juice
- 1 tablespoon capers, drained
- ½ tablespoon nutritional yeast
- ½ teaspoon Dijon mustard
- 2 medium garlic cloves
- ½ teaspoon salt
- ⅛ teaspoon freshly ground black pepper

METHOD

1. Put all the ingredients in a high-speed blender and blend until smooth and creamy.
2. Chill for at least 30 minutes before serving.
3. Refrigerate leftovers in an airtight container for up to a week.

*Note:
If you don't have a high-speed blender, soak the cashews in hot water for 15 minutes prior to blending. Discard soaking water and proceed as directed.

NUTRITIONAL INFORMATION (PER SERVING)

Per serving: Calories 98.9, Carbohydrate 6.4 g, Fiber 0.9 g, Total Sugars 1.2 g, Added Sugars 0 g, Fat 7.3 g, Saturated Fat 1.3 g, Protein 3.6 g, Sodium 394.9 mg, Iron 1.3 mg

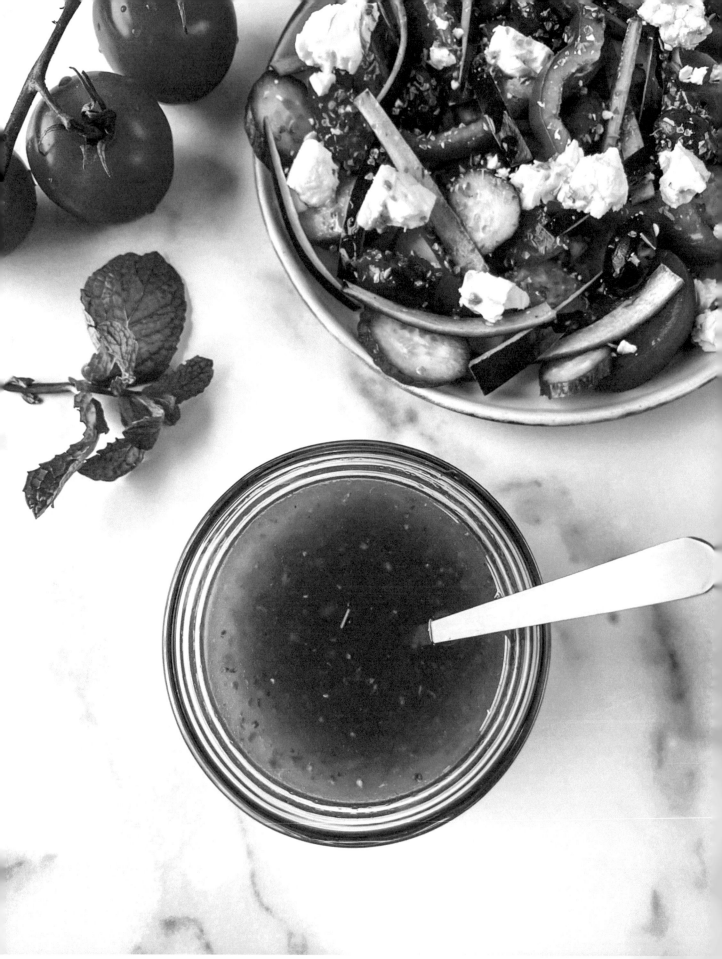

Greek Vinaigrette

Makes about 4 servings

This bright and tangy dressing is made with extra-virgin olive oil, fresh lemon juice, and red wine vinegar. Perfect for a classic Greek salad or drizzled over chilled whole-grain pasta with cucumbers, tomatoes, and fresh basil. This Greek Vinaigrette also makes an ideal marinade for chickpeas, cannellini beans, tofu, or roasted beets.

INGREDIENTS

- 6 tablespoons extra-virgin olive oil
- 2 tablespoons fresh lemon juice
- 1 tablespoon red wine vinegar
- 1 ½ teaspoons dried oregano
- 1 teaspoon pure maple syrup
- 2 medium garlic cloves, minced
- ½ teaspoon salt, or to taste
- ⅛ teaspoon freshly ground black pepper

METHOD

1. Place all ingredients in a pint-sized canning jar. Cover tightly and shake until fully emulsified.
2. Serve cold or at room temperature.
3. Refrigerate in an airtight container for up to 7 days.

Note:
The olive oil will solidify once refrigerated. To liquify, set on the counter for 10 minutes or run the jar under warm water for a couple of minutes and shake well.

NUTRITIONAL INFORMATION (PER SERVING)

Per serving: Calories 189.9, Carbohydrate 2.7 g, Fiber 0.2 g, Total Sugars 1.3 g, Added Sugars 1 g, Fat 20.3 g, Saturated Fat 2.8 g, Protein 0.2 g, Sodium 296.1 mg, Iron 0.3 mg

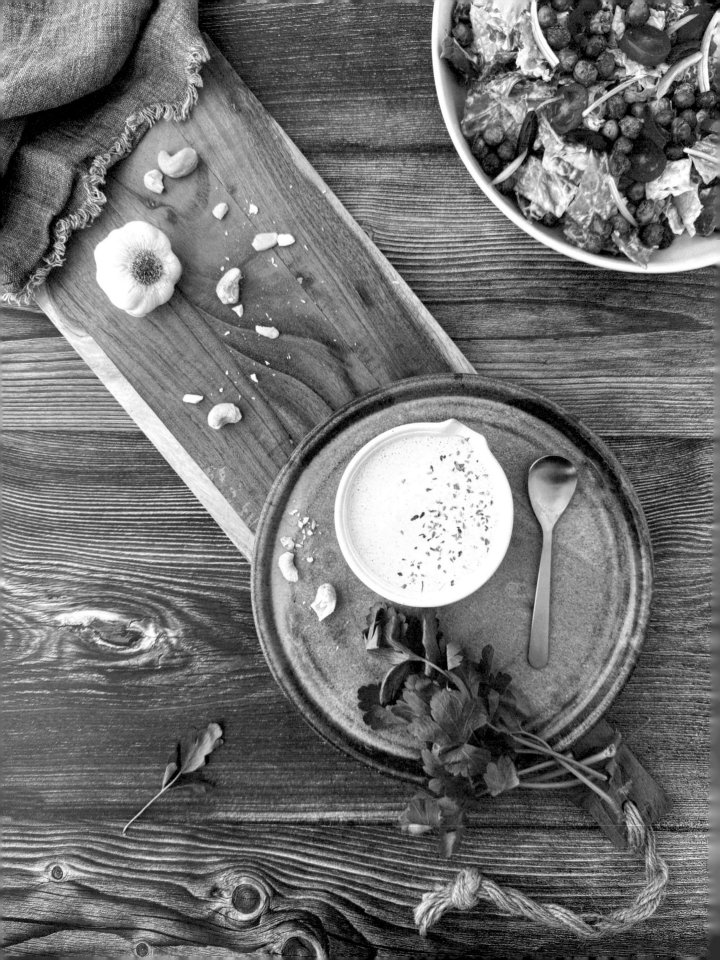

Creamy Greek Dressing

Makes about 4 servings

This tangy cashew-based creamy dressing is perfect for a Greek chopped salad or a Mediterranean chilled noodle salad loaded with raw veggies and herbs.

INGREDIENTS

- ½ cup raw cashews, *see note**
- ½ cup water
- 1 ½ tablespoons red wine vinegar
- 1 medium garlic clove
- 1 teaspoon dried oregano
- ½ teaspoon pure maple syrup
- ½ teaspoon Dijon mustard
- ½ teaspoon salt

METHOD

1. Put all the ingredients in a high-speed blender and blend until smooth and creamy.
2. Chill for at least 30 minutes before serving.
3. Refrigerate leftovers in an airtight container for up to a week.

*Note:
If you don't have a high-speed blender, soak the cashews in hot water for 15 minutes prior to blending. Discard soaking water and proceed as directed.

NUTRITIONAL INFORMATION (PER SERVING)

Per serving: Calories 95.5, Carbohydrate 5.9 g, Fiber 0.7 g, Total Sugars 1.5 g, Added Sugars 0.5 g, Fat 7.2 g, Saturated Fat 1.3 g, Protein 3.1 g, Sodium 313.6 mg, Iron 1.2 mg

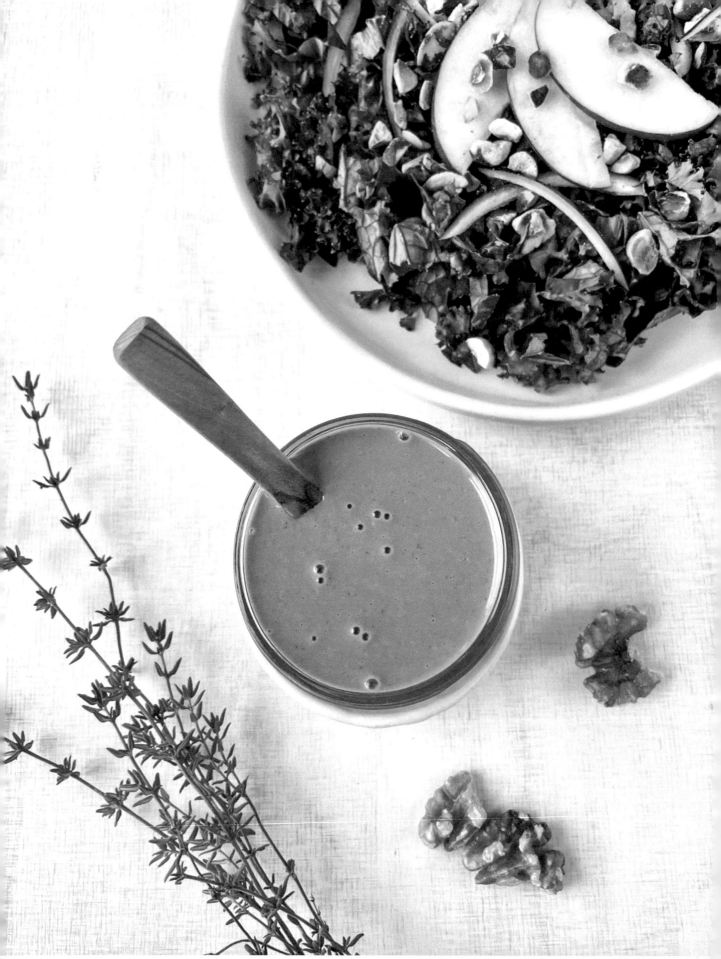

Balsamic Walnut Dressing

Makes about 4 servings

This oil-free dressing uses raw walnuts and aged balsamic vinegar to create a slightly sweet, tangy, and earthy dressing. It pairs beautifully with a mixed green salad topped with fresh fruit, like apples or strawberries, along with red onion and toasted pecans.

INGREDIENTS

- ¼ cup aged balsamic vinegar
- ⅓ cup raw walnut pieces
- ¼ cup water
- 1 tablespoon fresh lime juice
- ½ tablespoon Dijon mustard
- ½ tablespoon pure maple syrup
- 1 medium garlic clove
- ½ teaspoon dried thyme
- ¼ teaspoon salt
- ⅛ teaspoon freshly ground black pepper

METHOD

1. Put all the ingredients in a high-speed blender and blend until smooth and creamy.
2. Serve cold or at room temperature.
3. Refrigerate leftovers in an airtight container for up to a week.

NUTRITIONAL INFORMATION (PER SERVING)

Per serving: Calories 96.6, Carbohydrate 8.2 g, Fiber 0.9 g, Total Sugars 5.6 g, Added Sugars 1.5 g, Fat 6.4 g, Saturated Fat 0.6 g, Protein 1.8 g, Sodium 199.5 g, Iron 0.7 mg

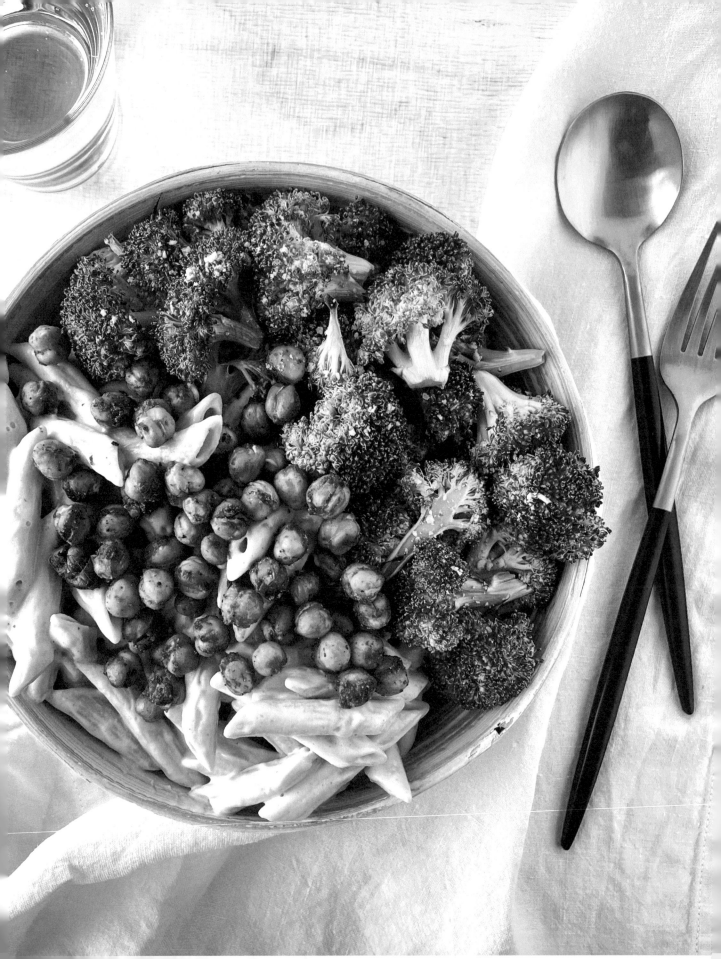

Alfredo Sauce

Makes about 4 servings

Combine this dairy-free alfredo sauce with your favorite whole-grain or legume pasta and top with roasted chickpeas and broccoli for a comforting bowl of yumminess!

INGREDIENTS

- 1 small white onion, chopped
- 1 cup low-sodium vegetable broth
- 4 medium garlic cloves, chopped
- ½ cup raw cashews, *see note**
- ⅓ cup water
- 2 tablespoons nutritional yeast
- 1 ½ tablespoons fresh lemon juice
- ½ teaspoon salt

*Note:
If you don't have a high-speed blender, soak the cashews in hot water for 15 minutes prior to blending. Discard soaking water and proceed as directed.

METHOD

1. Put the onions and broth in a saucepan over medium heat and cook until all the broth has evaporated, about 10 minutes, stirring frequently toward the end of the timing. Reduce heat if the onions start to burn.
2. Add the garlic and cook until fragrant, about a minute.
3. Transfer to a high-speed blender along with the remaining ingredients. Blend until smooth and creamy.
4. Taste and season with more salt and pepper, if desired.
5. Stir into 8 ounces of warm cooked pasta and vegetables.

NUTRITIONAL INFORMATION (PER SERVING)

Per serving: Calories 115.3, Carbohydrate 9.4 g, Fiber 1.4 g, Total Sugars 2.2 g, Added Sugars 0.3 g, Fat 7.2 g, Saturated Fat 1.3 g, Protein 4 g, Sodium 337.5 mg, Iron 1.4 mg

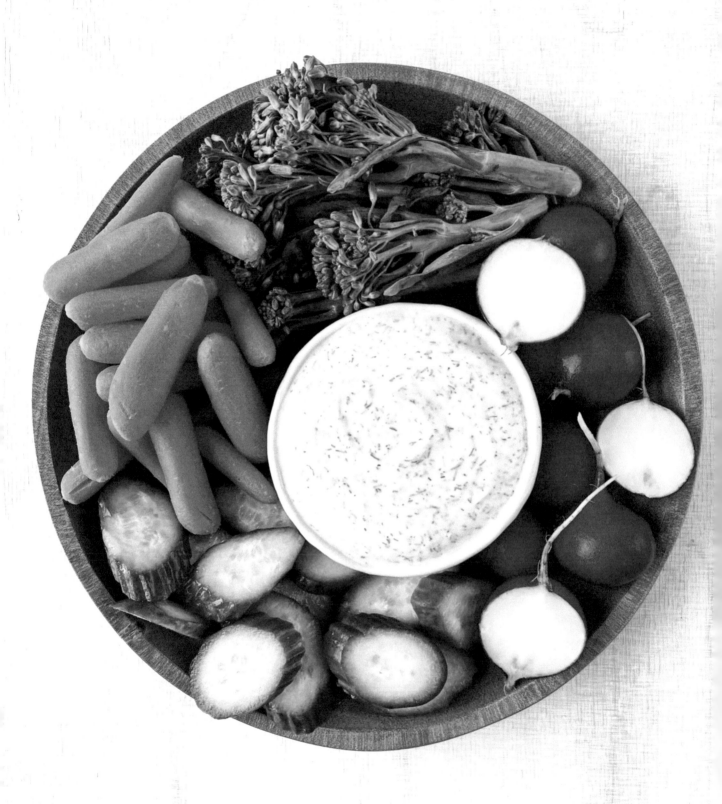

Dill Sauce

Makes about 4 servings

This yogurt sauce is my go-to for drizzling over buffalo wraps, Mediterranean-inspired pita sandwiches, and nourish bowls. Dill Sauce also makes a yummy dip for roasted and raw veggies.

INGREDIENTS

METHOD

- ½ cup plain, unsweetened cashew yogurt (or plain coconut yogurt)
- 1 tablespoon runny tahini
- 1 teaspoon dried dill (or 1 tablespoon fresh dill, minced)
- 1 medium garlic clove, minced (or ½ teaspoon garlic powder)
- 1 teaspoon white wine vinegar
- ½ teaspoon Dijon mustard
- ¼ teaspoon salt

1. Combine all the ingredients in a small bowl and stir.
2. Serve cold.
3. Refrigerate leftovers in an airtight container for up to a week.

NUTRITIONAL INFORMATION (PER SERVING)

Per serving: Calories 48.5, Carbohydrate 3.1 g, Fiber 0.6 g, Total Sugars 0.4 g, Added Sugars 0 g, Fat 3.6 g, Saturated Fat 0.5 g, Protein 1.5 g, Sodium 169.3 mg, Iron 0.6 mg

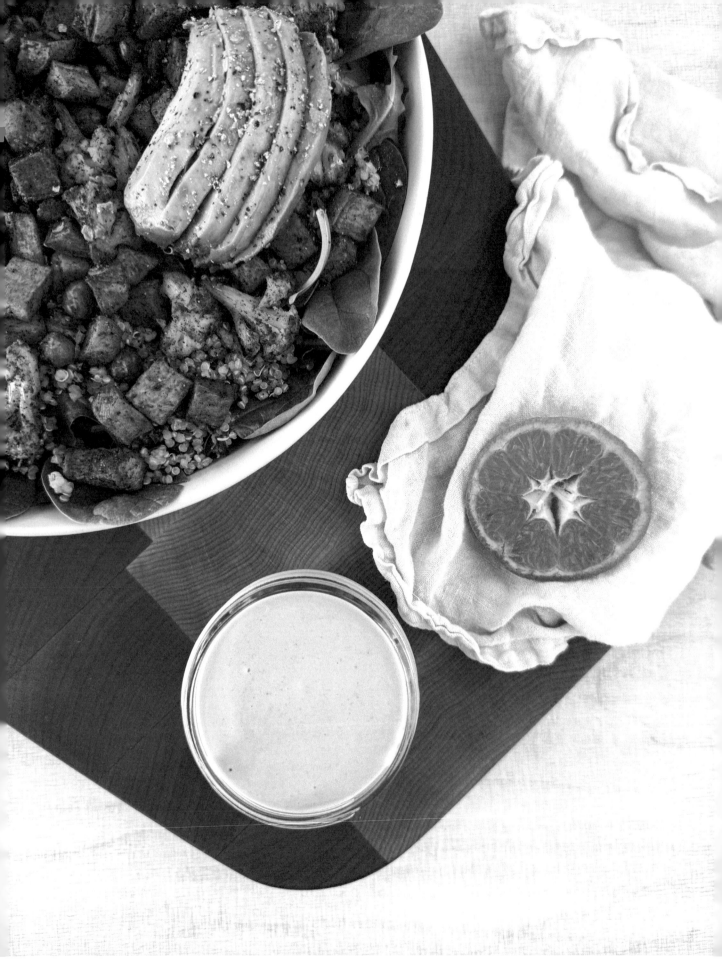

Citrus Tahini Sauce

Makes about 4 servings

This bright and earthy sauce is made with fresh citrus juice, tahini, and Dijon. Pairs well with Garlic Paprika Tofu Cubes (page 117) and seasonal roasted vegetables on a salad or in a nourish bowl.

INGREDIENTS

- ¼ cup tahini
- 3 tablespoons fresh orange juice (or lime juice, lemon juice, or a combination)
- 1 tablespoon rice vinegar
- ½ tablespoon Dijon mustard
- ½ tablespoon pure maple syrup
- 1 medium garlic clove, minced (or ½ teaspoon garlic powder)
- Ice-water as needed

METHOD

1. Put the tahini and orange juice in a medium bowl. Whisk together until smooth and creamy.
2. Add the rice vinegar, Dijon, maple syrup, and garlic and whisk until combined. If the dressing is too thick, add a teaspoon of ice-cold water at a time until you reach a pourable consistency. This will depend on how runny the tahini is.
3. Serve cold or at room temperature.
4. Refrigerate leftovers in an airtight container for up to 7 days.

NUTRITIONAL INFORMATION (PER SERVING)

Per serving: Calories 109, Carbohydrate 4.8 g, Fiber 1.3 g, Total Sugars 2.4 g, Added Sugars 1.5 g, Fat 9.4 g, Saturated Fat 1.1 g, Protein 3.1 g, Sodium 25.1 mg, Iron 1.1 mg

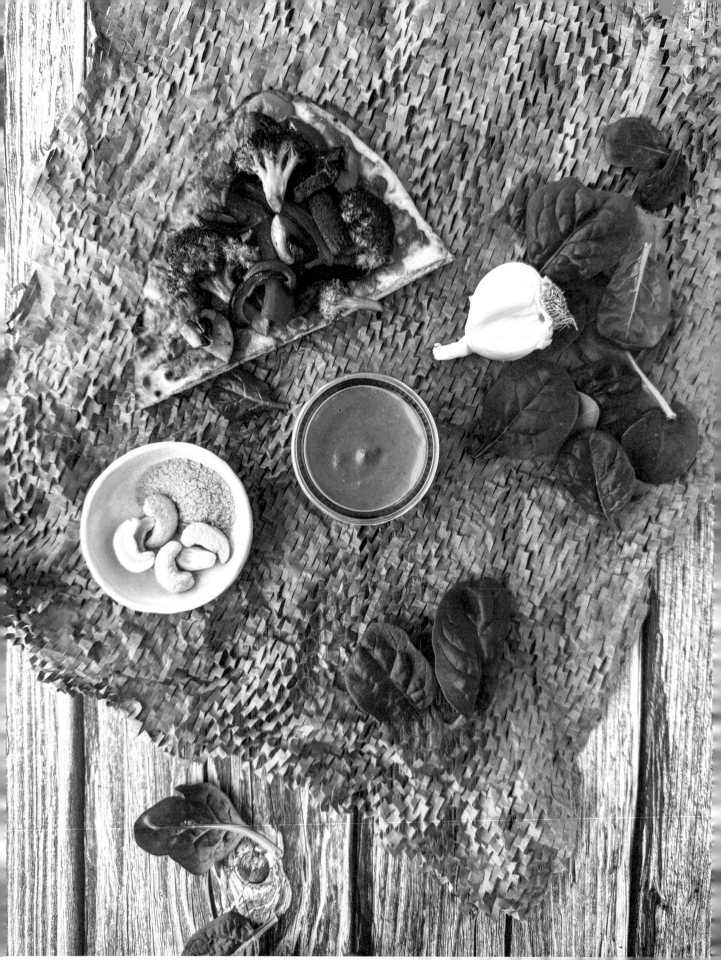

Basil Spinach Pesto

Makes about 8 servings

This Basil Spinach Pesto pairs perfectly with roasted vegetables and whole-grain pasta. For a flavor and nutrient boost, try swapping out mayonnaise with this vibrant pesto on wraps and sandwiches.

INGREDIENTS

- 2 cups fresh basil leaves
- 2 cups fresh baby spinach, loosely packed
- ½ cup extra-virgin olive oil
- ¼ cup nutritional yeast
- ¼ cup raw cashews, *see note**
- 4 medium garlic cloves
- 2 tablespoons fresh lemon juice
- ¾ teaspoon salt, or to taste

METHOD

1. Put all the ingredients in a high-speed blender and blend until smooth and creamy.
2. Serve warm or cold.
3. Store in an airtight container and refrigerate for up to 5 days or freeze for up to 2 months.

VARIATIONS

1. Greens: Instead of spinach, use 2 cups fresh kale.
2. Nuts: Instead of cashews, use toasted pine nuts, pistachios, or hemp hearts.

*Note:
If you don't have a high-speed blender, soak the cashews in hot water for 15 minutes prior to blending. Discard soaking water and proceed as directed.

NUTRITIONAL INFORMATION (PER SERVING)

Per serving: Calories 159, Carbohydrate 3.5 g, Fiber 1 g, Total Sugars 0.4 g, Added Sugars 0 g, Fat 15.4 g, Saturated Fat 2.2 g, Protein 2.9 g, Sodium 233.5 mg, Iron 1.1 mg

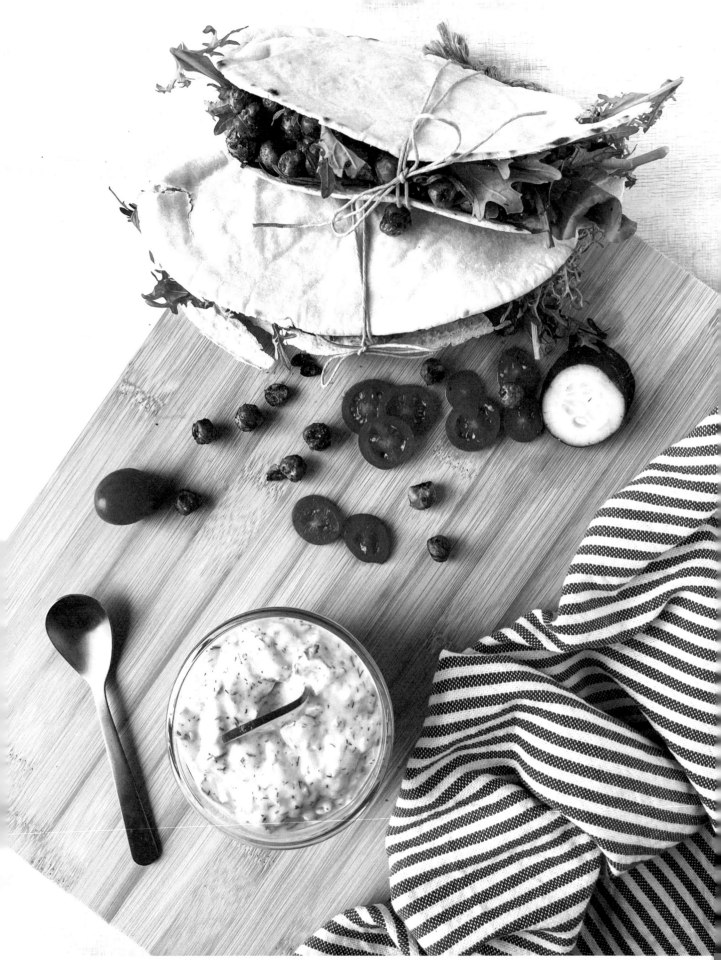

Tzatziki Sauce

Made with nondairy yogurt, cucumbers, and fresh dill, this Mediterranean-inspired sauce brings a cool, tangy finish to Greek pita sandwiches and nourish bowls. Or serve it as part of a fresh mezze platter with olives, whole-grain pita and seed crackers, cucumbers, grapes, tomatoes, radishes, and a handful of nuts.

INGREDIENTS

- ½ medium cucumber, unpeeled and grated
- ¾ cup plain, unsweetened cashew yogurt (or plain coconut yogurt)
- 1 tablespoon extra-virgin olive oil
- 1 tablespoon fresh lemon juice
- 1 medium garlic clove, minced
- 1 teaspoon dried dill (or 1 tablespoon fresh dill, minced)
- ¼ teaspoon salt, or to taste

METHOD

1. Put the grated cucumber on a tea towel and squeeze out excess liquid.
2. In a medium bowl, combine the cucumber, yogurt, oil, lemon juice, garlic, dill, and salt. Stir until well combined.
3. Serve cold.
4. Refrigerate leftovers in an airtight container for up to 7 days.

NUTRITIONAL INFORMATION (PER SERVING)

Per serving: Calories 35.7, Carbohydrate 2.2 g, Fiber 0.3 g, Total Sugars 0.4 g, Added Sugars 0 g, Fat 2.8 g, Saturated Fat 0.4 g, Protein 0.6 g, Sodium 75.6 mg, Iron 0.1 mg

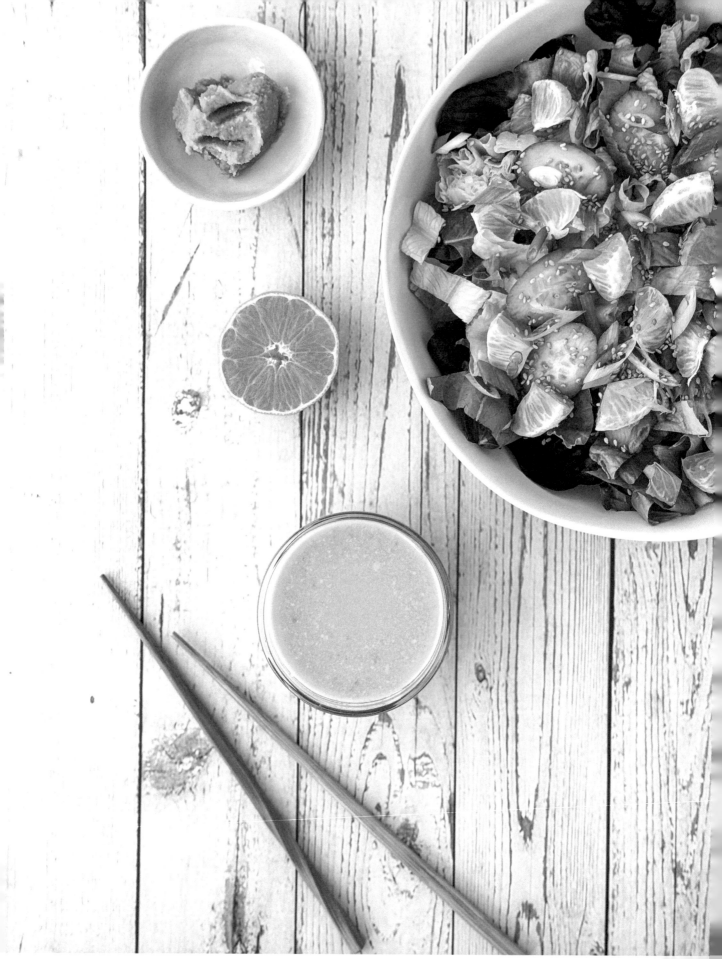

Mandarin Miso Dressing

Makes about 4 servings

Bright with citrus and umami flavors, Mandarin Miso Dressing is the perfect complement to a base of crunchy salads greens or chilled soba noodles topped with mandarin slices, sesame seeds, green onions, and cucumber.

INGREDIENTS

- 3 tablespoons white miso paste
- 2 tablespoons rice vinegar
- 1 tablespoon tahini
- 1 tablespoon water
- ¼ cup freshly juiced mandarin oranges (about 2 medium mandarins)
- 1 teaspoon toasted sesame oil
- 1 teaspoon maple syrup

METHOD

1. Combine the miso paste, rice vinegar, tahini, and water in a small bowl and briskly whisk together until smooth and creamy.
2. Add the mandarin juice, sesame oil, and maple syrup and whisk until combined.
3. Serve cold.
4. Refrigerate leftovers in an airtight container for up to 7 days.

NUTRITIONAL INFORMATION (PER SERVING)

Per serving: Calories 79.9, Carbohydrate 10 g, Fiber 1.5 g, Total Sugars 5.7 g, Added Sugars 1 g, Fat 3.3 g, Saturated Fat 0.5 g, Protein 2.5 g, Sodium 538.2 mg, Iron 0.4 mg

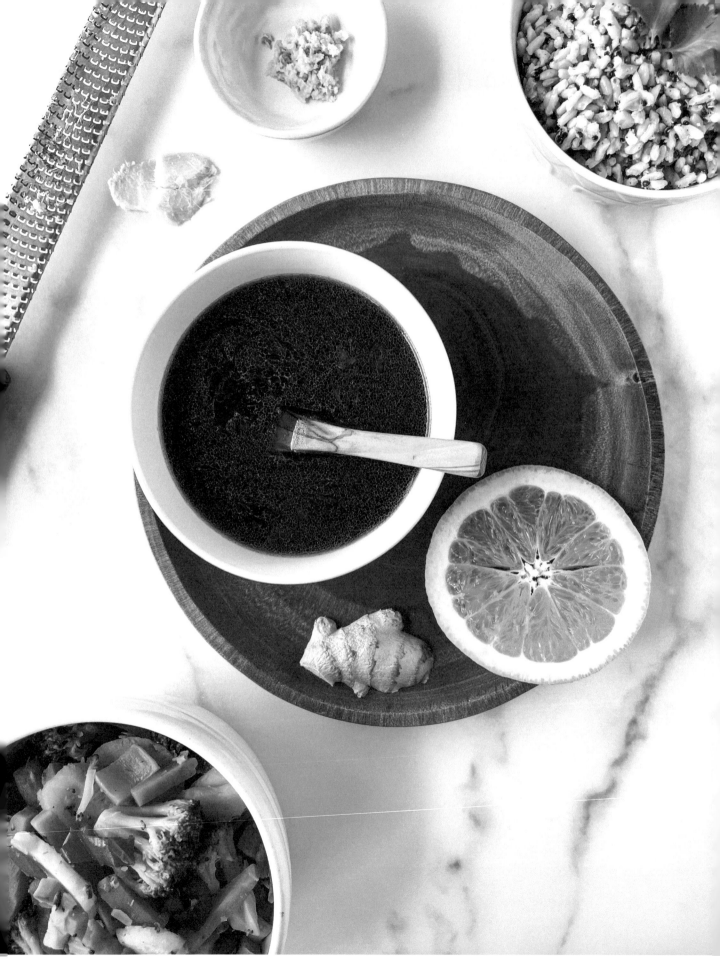

Orange Sesame Sauce

Makes about 6 servings

This versatile sauce is my go-to for Asian-inspired flavors. Drizzle it over crunchy cabbage salads, stir-fries, noodle bowls, or fried rice. Use it to marinate super-firm tofu or tempeh, or as a dipping sauce for fresh spring rolls, gyoza, or lettuce wraps

INGREDIENTS

- ¼ cup fresh orange juice (about 1 large navel orange)
- ¼ cup Tamari Lite
- 2 tablespoons fresh lime juice
- 1 tablespoon pure maple syrup
- 1 teaspoon toasted sesame oil
- 2 teaspoons minced fresh ginger
- 1 teaspoon sriracha, or to taste
- 1 medium garlic clove, minced

METHOD

1. Put all the ingredients in a pint-size jar and shake until combined.
2. Serve warm or cold.
3. Refrigerate leftovers in an airtight container for up to 7 days.

Variation:
Stir-fry sauce: In a small saucepan, whisk the prepared sauce with 2 teaspoons of arrowroot or cornstarch until smooth. Heat over medium heat until slightly thickened and warm. Pour over the stir-fry ingredients, toss to coat, and serve over brown rice.

NUTRITIONAL INFORMATION (PER SERVING)

Per serving: Calories 41, Carbohydrate 7.7 g, Fiber 0.8 g, Total Sugars 5.1 g, Added Sugars 2.1 g, Fat 0.8 g, Saturated Fat 0.1 g, Protein 1.1 g, Sodium 350.5 mg, Iron 0.8 mg

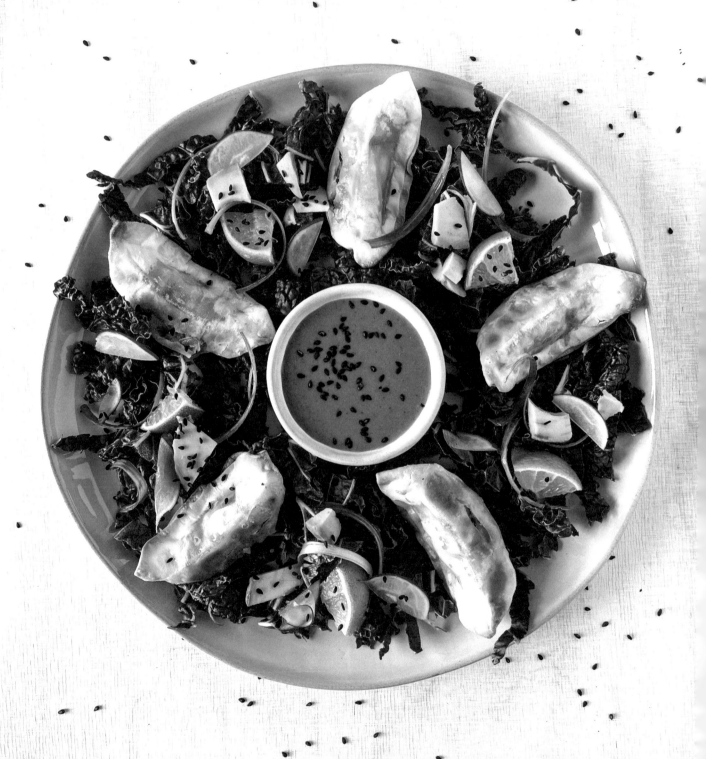

Peanut Ginger Sauce

Makes about 4 servings

This creamy and tangy peanut sauce is a key addition to stir-fries, and noodle bowls. Peanut Ginger Sauce also makes an excellent dipping sauce for tofu skewers and spring rolls.

INGREDIENTS

- 3 tablespoons smooth peanut butter, *see note**
- 2 tablespoons fresh lime juice
- 2 tablespoons Tamari Lite
- 1 tablespoon pure maple syrup
- ½ tablespoon toasted sesame oil
- 2 teaspoons sriracha
- 2 teaspoons minced fresh ginger
- 1 medium garlic clove, minced
- 2 tablespoons warm water, more as needed

METHOD

1. Whisk all the ingredients in a jar until well combined. Taste and adjust. Add more lime juice for acidity and more sriracha for heat. If the mixture is too thick, add a tablespoon more of water at a time until you reach a pourable consistency.
2. Serve warm or cold.
3. Refrigerate leftovers in an airtight container for up to 7 days.

*Note:
Peanut allergy:
Use almond butter,
cashew butter, or
sunflower butter.

NUTRITIONAL INFORMATION (PER SERVING)

Per serving: Calories 111.9, Carbohydrate 8.4 g, Fiber 1.2 g, Total Sugars 4.2 g, Added Sugars 3.4 g, Fat 7.8 g, Saturated Fat 1.2 g, Protein 3.6 g, Sodium 316.3 mg, Iron 0.9 mg

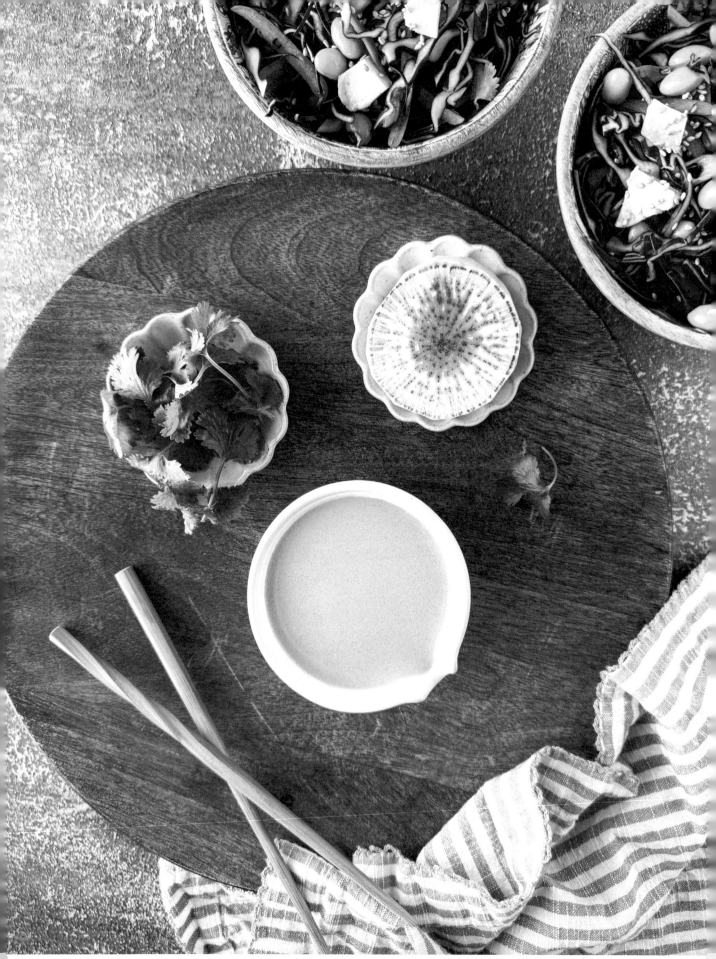

Sesame Ginger Dressing

Makes about 4 servings

This creamy Asian-inspired dressing is made with pantry ingredients and comes together in five minutes. Add it to crunchy cabbage salad or stir into warm soba noodles topped with shelled edamame, avocado, and toasted nuts.

INGREDIENTS

- 3 tablespoons tahini
- 2 tablespoons ice-cold water
- 3 tablespoons rice vinegar
- 1 tablespoon toasted sesame oil
- 1 tablespoon Tamari Lite
- 1 tablespoon pure maple syrup
- 2 teaspoons minced fresh ginger
- Cold water to desired consistency, optional

METHOD

1. In a small bowl, whisk the tahini, water, and vinegar until super smooth and creamy.
2. Add the sesame oil, tamari, maple syrup, and ginger, then whisk until well combined. If the mixture is too thick, gradually add a teaspoon of cold water until the sauce reaches a pourable consistency.
3. Serve warm or cold.
4. Refrigerate leftovers in an airtight container for up to 7 days.

NUTRITIONAL INFORMATION (PER SERVING)

Per serving: Calories 124, Carbohydrate 5.7 g, Fiber 1 g, Total Sugars 3.3 g, Added Sugars 3 g, Fat 10.5 g, Saturated Fat 1.5 g, Protein 2.8 g, Sodium 186 mg, Iron 1.3 mg

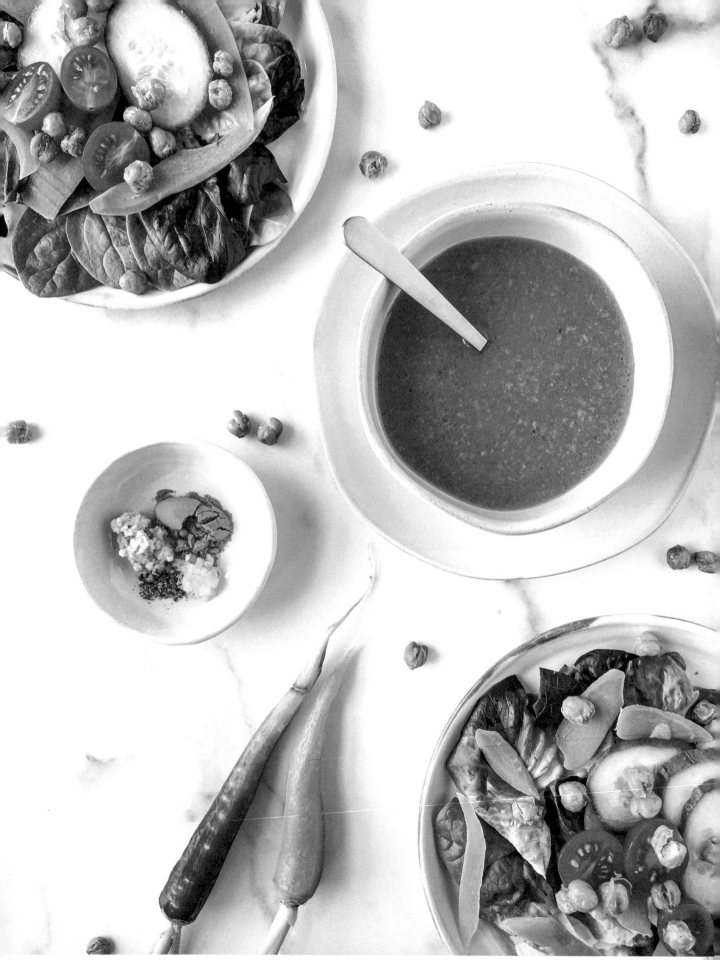

Ginger Turmeric Vinaigrette

Makes about 4 servings

Bright and earthy, this vinaigrette combines extra-virgin olive oil, turmeric powder, and fresh ginger for a delightful burst of flavor. Ginger Turmeric Vinaigrette pairs well with Mediterranean-, Indian-, and American-inspired salads. Drizzle over roasted vegetables, beans, or whole grains for a punch of flavor.

INGREDIENTS

- 6 tablespoons extra-virgin olive oil
- 2 tablespoons raw apple cider vinegar
- ½ tablespoon pure maple syrup
- ½ tablespoon Dijon mustard
- 2 teaspoons minced fresh ginger
- ½ teaspoon ground turmeric
- ¼ teaspoon salt
- ⅛ teaspoon freshly ground black pepper

METHOD

1. Put all the ingredients in a pint-size canning jar. Cover and shake until all the ingredients have emulsified. Taste and season with additional salt if desired.
2. Serve cold or at room temperature.
3. Refrigerate leftovers in an airtight container for up to 7 days.

Note:
The olive oil will solidify once refrigerated. To liquify, set on the counter for 10 minutes or run the jar under warm water for a couple of minutes and shake well.

NUTRITIONAL INFORMATION (PER SERVING)

Per serving: Calories 191.4, Carbohydrate 2.7 g, Fiber 0.2 g, Total Sugars 1.6 g, Added Sugars 1.5 g, Fat 20.4 g, Saturated Fat 2.8 g, Protein 0.2 g, Sodium 193.6 mg, Iron 0.4 mg

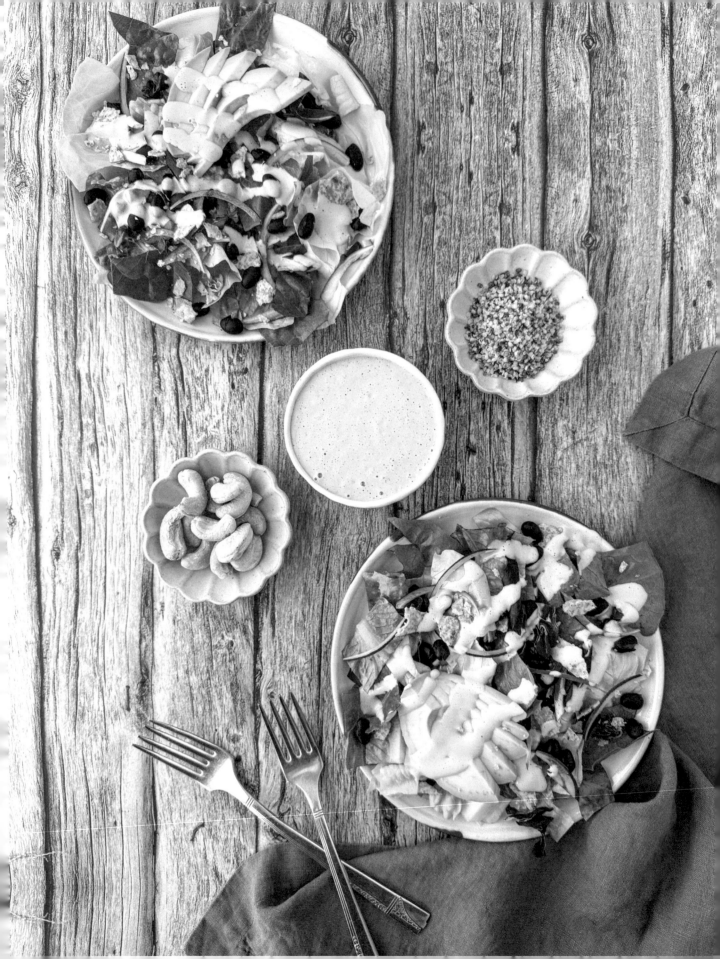

Creamy Cilantro Dressing

Makes about 4 servings

This vibrant and creamy dressing, made with cashews, hemp hearts, and fresh cilantro, is a perfect match for a Southwest-style salad or nourish bowl. Enjoy it with toppings like black beans, sweet corn, bell pepper, red onion, avocado, and crumbled corn tortilla chips.

INGREDIENTS

- ¼ cup raw cashews, *see note**
- ¼ cup hemp hearts, *see note**
- ½ cup water
- ½ cup fresh cilantro (leaves and some stems)
- 2 tablespoons fresh lime juice
- ¼ small (about ½-inch piece) jalapeño, seeds and ribs removed
- ½ teaspoon garlic powder
- ½ teaspoon onion powder
- ½ teaspoon pure maple syrup
- ½ teaspoon salt, or to taste

METHOD

1. Put all the ingredients in a high-speed blender and blend until smooth and creamy.
2. Chill for at least 30 minutes before serving.
3. Refrigerate leftovers in an airtight container for up to 5 days.

*Note:
If you don't have
a high-speed blender,
soak the cashews in hot water
for 15 minutes prior to blending.
Discard soaking water and proceed
as directed.

If you have a tree nut allergy, you
can omit the cashews and use
an additional ¼ cup of
hemp hearts.

NUTRITIONAL INFORMATION (PER SERVING)

Per serving: Calories 323.9, Carbohydrate 8.8 g, Fiber 3 g, Total Sugars 2 g, Added Sugars 0.5 g, Fat 23.2 g, Saturated Fat 2.8 g, Protein 14.4 g, Sodium 301.7 mg, Iron 2.6 mg

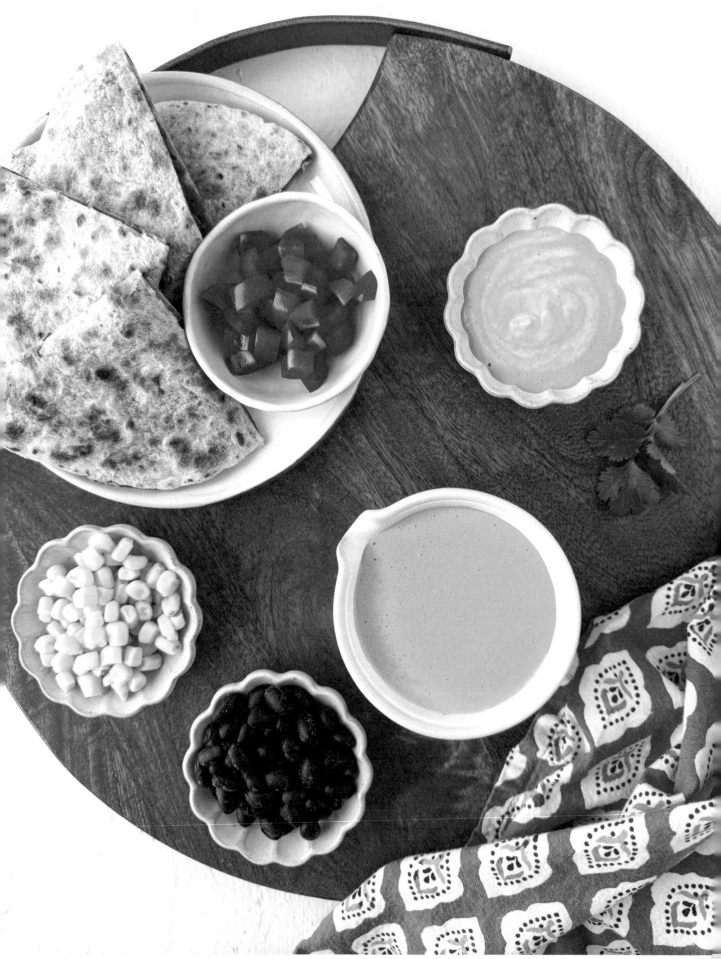

Cashew Queso

Makes about 8 servings

When Ted and I transitioned to a plant-forward diet, we missed cheese! This Cashew Queso is our go-to cheese sauce for all things Mexican. Drizzle it over sheet pan nachos, tacos, burritos, tostadas, enchiladas, and fajitas. Serve it as a delicious appetizer with corn tortilla chips and Pico de Gallo (page 81).

INGREDIENTS

- ½ cup raw cashews, *see note**
- ½ cup hot water
- 1 ½ tablespoons nutritional yeast
- 1 tablespoon Frank's RedHot Original Cayenne Pepper Sauce
- ½ teaspoon garlic powder
- ¼ teaspoon onion powder
- ¼ teaspoon ground turmeric
- ¼ teaspoon salt

METHOD

1. Put all the ingredients in a high-speed blender and blend until smooth and creamy.
2. Serve warm or at room temperature.
3. Refrigerate leftovers in an airtight container for up to 7 days.

*Note:
If you don't have a high-speed blender, soak the cashews in hot water for 15 minutes prior to blending. Discard soaking water and proceed as directed.

NUTRITIONAL INFORMATION (PER SERVING)

Per serving: Calories 49.9, Carbohydrate 3.1 g, Fiber 0.5 g, Total Sugars 0.5 g, Added Sugars 0 g, Fat 3.6 g, Saturated Fat 0.6 g, Protein 2.1 g, Sodium 148.6 mg, Iron 0.7 mg

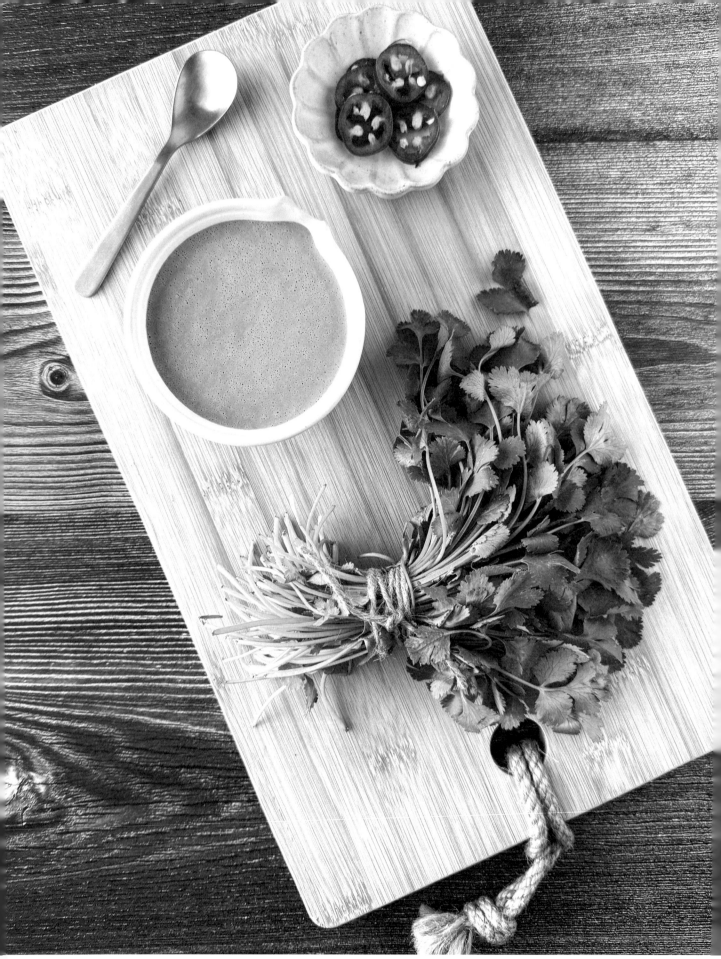

Cilantro Lime Crema

Makes about 6 servings

This herby, cashew-based sauce is bursting with flavor! Skip the cheese and drizzle this delicious sauce over your favorite Mexican dishes.

INGREDIENTS

- ⅓ cup raw cashews, *see note**
- ¼ cup water
- ¼ small jalapeño, ribs and seeds removed
- 1 cup fresh cilantro (leaves and some stems)
- 2 tablespoons fresh lime juice
- 1 medium garlic clove
- ½ teaspoon salt
- ¼ teaspoon cumin

METHOD

1. Put all the ingredients in a high-speed blender and blend until smooth and creamy.
2. Serve cold or at room temperature.
3. Refrigerate leftovers in an airtight container for up to 4 days.

*Note:
If you don't have a high-speed blender, soak the cashews in hot water for 15 minutes prior to blending. Discard soaking water and proceed as directed.

If you don't like cilantro, feel free to omit.

NUTRITIONAL INFORMATION (PER SERVING)

Per serving: Calories 42.6, Carbohydrate 2.9 g, Fiber 0.4 g, Total Sugars 0.6 g, Added Sugars 0 g, Fat 3.2 g, Saturated Fat 0.6 g, Protein 1.4 g, Sodium 199.3 mg, Iron 0.6 mg

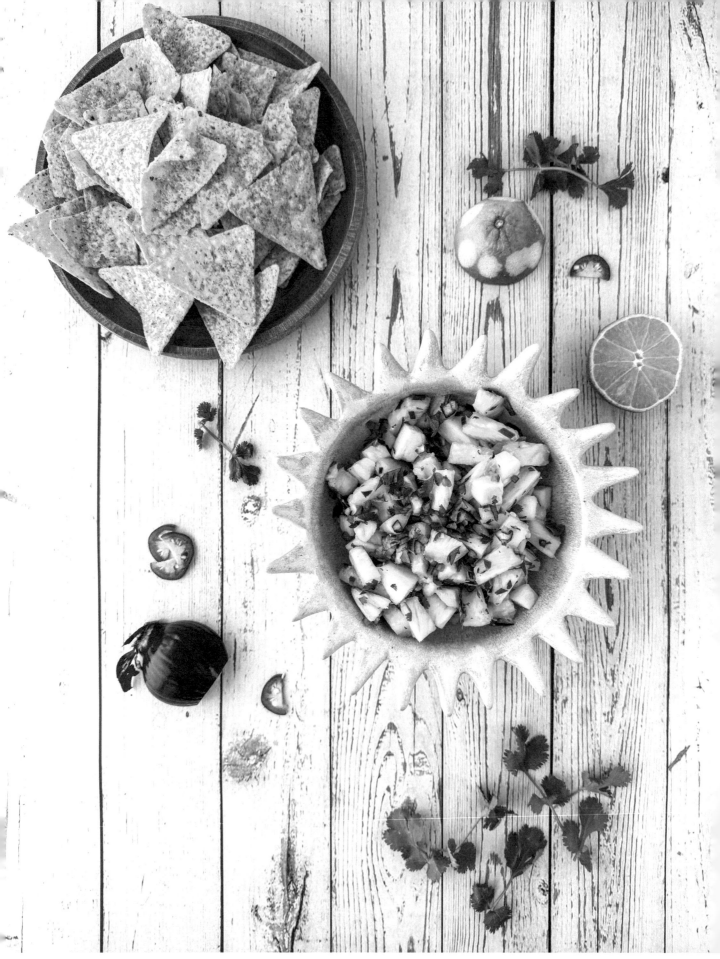

Pineapple Salsa

Makes about 8 servings

This bright and zesty salsa blends fresh pineapple with jalapeño, onion, and cilantro. Ideal for adding a burst of flavor to Caribbean- and Latin-inspired tacos or nourish bowls. It also makes a delicious appetizer with tortilla chips.

INGREDIENTS

- ½ medium pineapple, peeled, cored, and diced
- ½ small jalapeño, minced (seeds and ribs removed)
- 2 tablespoons finely diced red onion
- ⅓ cup chopped fresh cilantro leaves
- 2 tablespoons fresh lime juice
- Zest of ½ lime
- ¼ teaspoon salt

METHOD

1. Combine all the ingredients in a medium bowl.
2. Refrigerate leftovers in an airtight container for up to 4 days.

NUTRITIONAL INFORMATION (PER SERVING)

Per serving: Calories 30.8, Carbohydrate 8.1 g, Fiber 0.9 g, Total Sugars 5.8 g, Added Sugars 0 g, Fat 0.1 g, Saturated Fat 0 g, Protein 0.4 g, Sodium 74.8 mg, Iron 0.2 mg

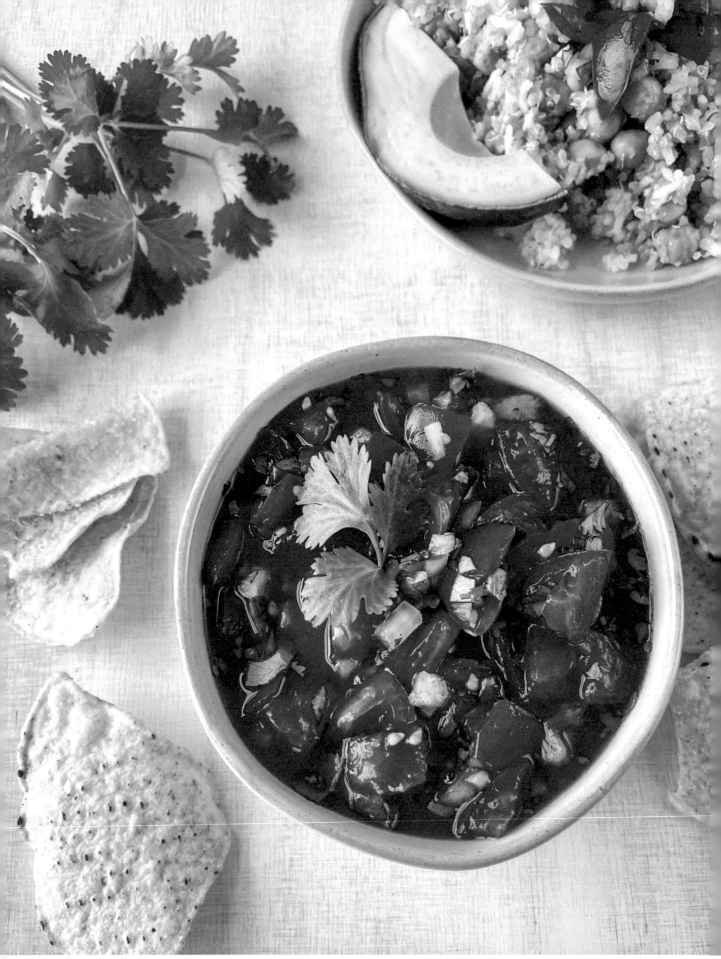

Pico de Gallo

Makes about 8 servings

This chunky salsa, made with ripe tomatoes, onion, and cilantro, adds brightness and texture to your favorite Mexican dishes, or serve with tortilla chips as an appetizer.

INGREDIENTS

- 10 ounces ripe tomatoes, finely diced
- ⅓ cup finely diced white onion
- 2 tablespoons fresh lime juice
- ½ cup firmly packed fresh cilantro leaves, chopped
- ¼ teaspoon salt

METHOD

1. Combine all the ingredients in a medium bowl and gently toss.
2. Refrigerate in an airtight container for up to 4 days.

NUTRITIONAL INFORMATION (PER SERVING)

Per serving: Calories 10.7, Carbohydrate 2.5 g, Fiber 0.6 g, Total Sugars 1.3 g, Added Sugars 0 g, Fat 0.1 g, Saturated Fat 0 g, Protein 0.4 g, Sodium 76.3 mg, Iron 0.1 mg

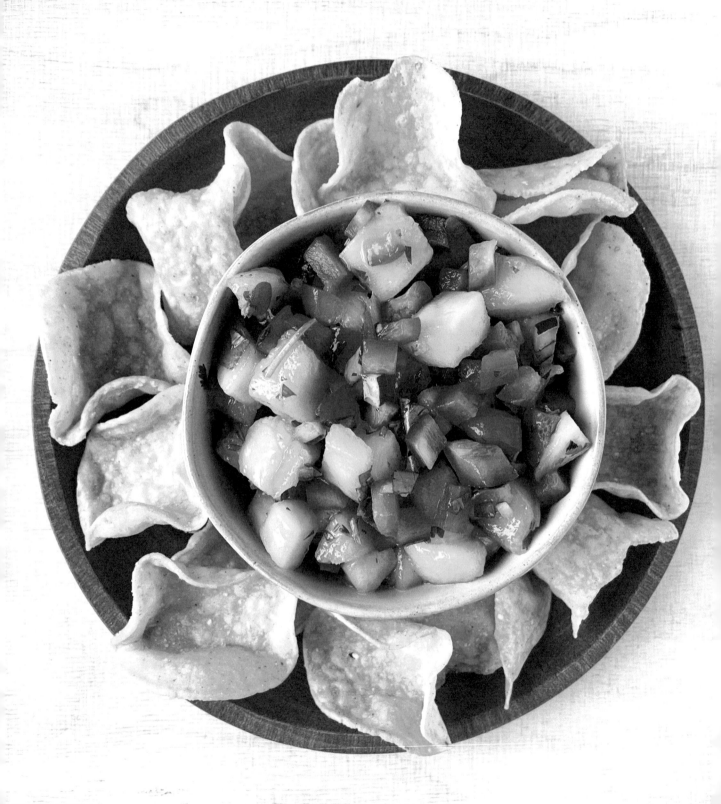

Mango Salsa

Sweet, ripe mango is mixed with red bell pepper, jalapeño, red onion, lime juice, and cilantro for a colorful and refreshing salsa. Perfect as a topping for Mexican dishes or served as a tasty appetizer with tortilla chips.

INGREDIENTS

- 1 large ripe mango, peeled, pitted, and diced
- ½ medium red bell pepper, diced
- ¼ cup finely diced red onion
- 1 tablespoon minced jalapeño (seeds and ribs removed)
- ⅓ cup chopped fresh cilantro leaves
- 1 tablespoon fresh lime, mandarin, or orange juice
- ¼ teaspoon salt

METHOD

1. Combine all the ingredients in a medium bowl and stir.
2. Refrigerate leftovers in an airtight container for up to 4 days.

NUTRITIONAL INFORMATION (PER SERVING)

Per serving: Calories 60.9, Carbohydrate 15.1 g, Fiber 1.9 g, Total Sugars 12.8 g, Added Sugars 0 g, Fat 0.4 g, Saturated Fat 0.1 g, Protein 1 g, Sodium 149.9 mg, Iron 0.3 mg

VEGETABLES

Raw + Cooked

Vegetables add vibrant color to your plate, and that color is a sign of the antioxidants, vitamins, and minerals they contain—all essential for a healthy gut and a happy heart. Aim to fill half your plate with vegetables at lunch and dinner to maximize nutrition and flavor!

- Roasted Vegetable Chart
- Raw Rainbow Veggie Toppers
- Garlic Miso Mushrooms
- Balsamic Brussels Sprouts
- Roasted Asparagus
- Sautéed Broccoli
- Sautéed Bell Peppers
- Massaged Kale Salad with Apples
- Mushroom Walnut Taco Filling

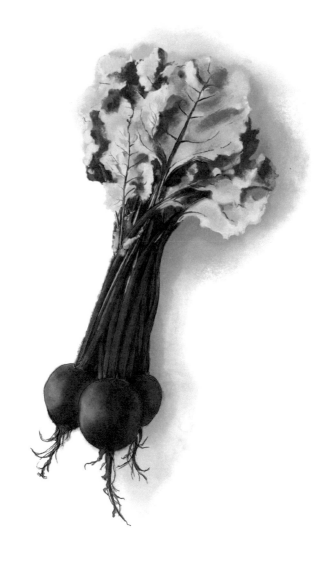

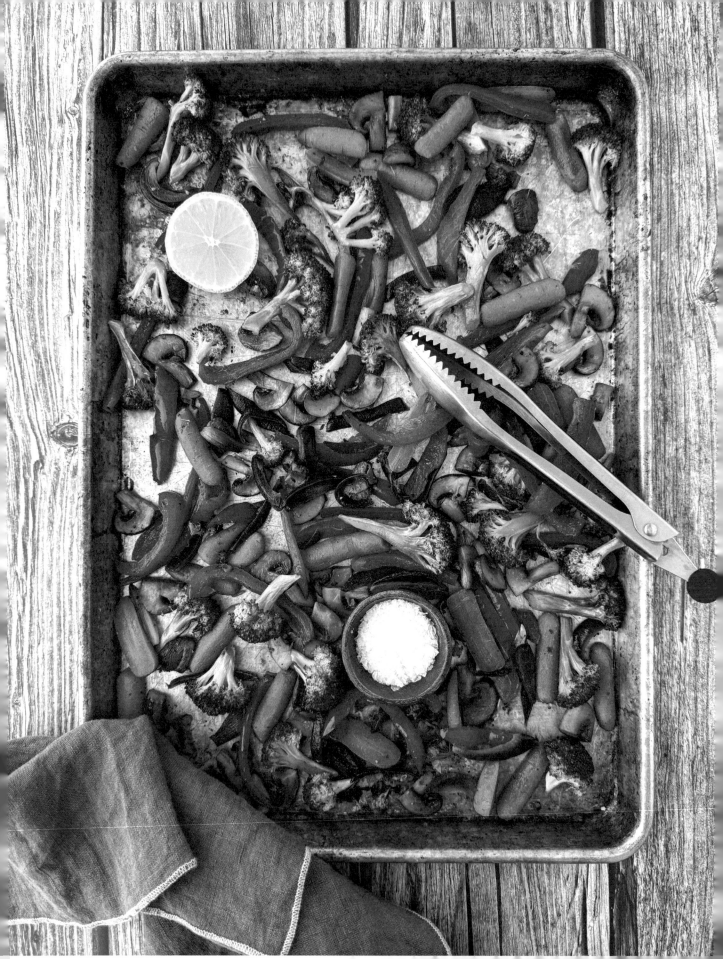

Roasted Vegetables Chart

Estimated Cook Times in Minutes

Asparagus, ends trimmed .... 6–10 mins

Beets, ½-inch cubes .... 30–40 mins

Bell peppers, ½-inch slices ....15–20 mins

Broccoli, florets .... 15–20 mins

Brussels sprouts, quartered ....15–20 mins

Butternut squash, ½-inch cubes .... 25–30 mins

Carrots, 1-inch diagonal pieces .... 20–25 mins

Cauliflower, florets .... 25–30 mins

Mushrooms, quartered
(button + baby bella) .... 13–18 mins

Onions, ½-inch slices .... 15–20 mins

Potatoes, ½-inch cubes .... 25–35 mins

Sweet potatoes, ½-inch cubes .... 25–35 mins

Tomatoes (cherry or grape) .... 15–25 mins

Zucchini, ½-inch half moons .... 15 mins

FLAVOR + NUTRIENT BOOSTERS

- Dried herbs + spices (add before cooking): For extra flavor, stir in your favorite dried spices to taste. Great options include garlic powder, oregano, thyme, cumin, paprika, or chili powder.

- Fresh herbs (add after cooking): For extra flavor and texture, add freshly chopped tender herbs just before serving, to taste. Great options include parsley, mint, dill, chives, or cilantro.

- Acid (add after cooking): For added brightness, stir in 1 tablespoon of lemon or lime juice or a drizzle of aged balsamic vinegar.

- Eat the rainbow: For nutrient diversity, cook a variety of veggies together at the same time. Yummy combinations include cauliflower, carrots, and potatoes, or asparagus, bell pepper, and zucchini.

METHOD

1. Preheat oven to 425°F. Line one or two rimmed baking sheets with parchment paper.

2. Wash, dry, and cut 1 pound of vegetables into even pieces.

3. Place the vegetables on a baking sheet and drizzle with 1 tablespoon of extra-virgin olive oil and a pinch of salt. Toss until evenly coated. Arrange in a single layer to ensure even cooking. If the vegetables are too crowded, use the second baking sheet.

4. Roast on the middle oven rack for the suggested time, stirring halfway through until golden and tender. Ovens vary, so keep an eye on your veggies and adjust the cooking time and temperature as needed for best results.

5. Season with additional salt and pepper, if desired.

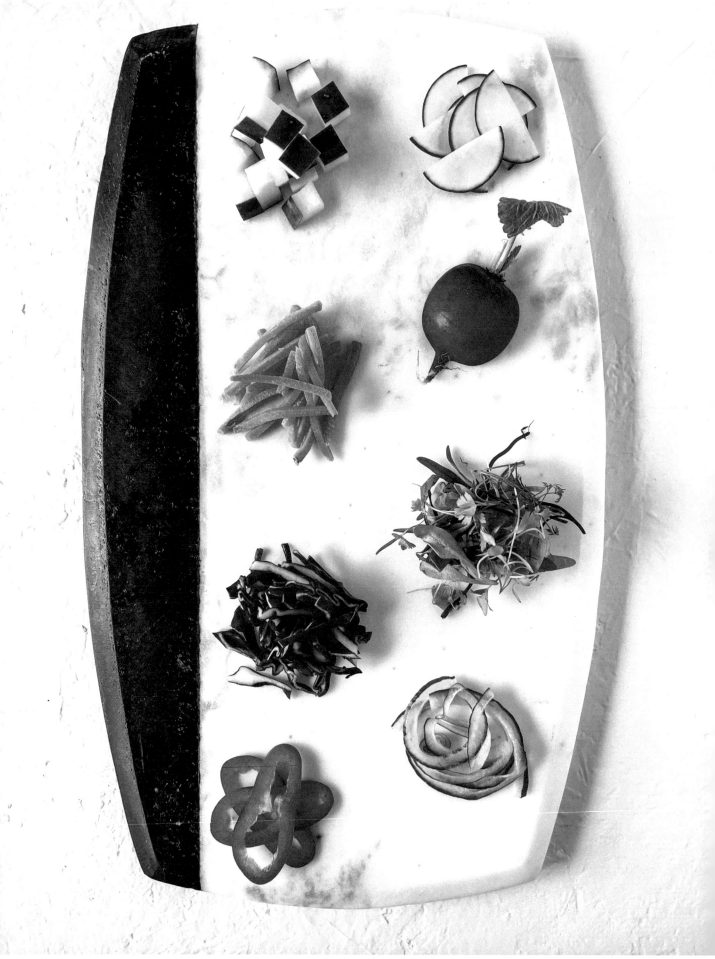

Raw Rainbow Veggie Toppers

Boost the color, fiber, and texture of your nourish bowls, salads, tacos, and wraps with veggie and fruit toppers. Choose one or more ingredients to add to each meal, as desired.

MEAL-PREP-FRIENDLY TOPPERS

- Beets, diced or sliced
- Cabbage, thinly sliced (red or green)
- Celery, diced
- Fennel, thinly sliced
- Fermented veggies
- Green onions, thinly sliced
- Pickled ginger
- Radish, thinly sliced or matchsticks
- Red onion, diced or thinly sliced

Tip:
Opt for pre-prepped options like matchstick carrots or bagged cabbage slaw to save time.

METHOD

1. Chop and store these ingredients in an airtight container for easy use throughout the week.

JUST BEFORE-SERVING TOPPERS

For the freshest flavor and texture, prepare just before serving.
- Avocado, diced or sliced
- Bell peppers, diced or sliced (red, yellow, orange, green)
- Fresh herbs, chopped or torn (parsley, basil, dill, cilantro, chives)
- Microgreens
- Tomatoes, diced

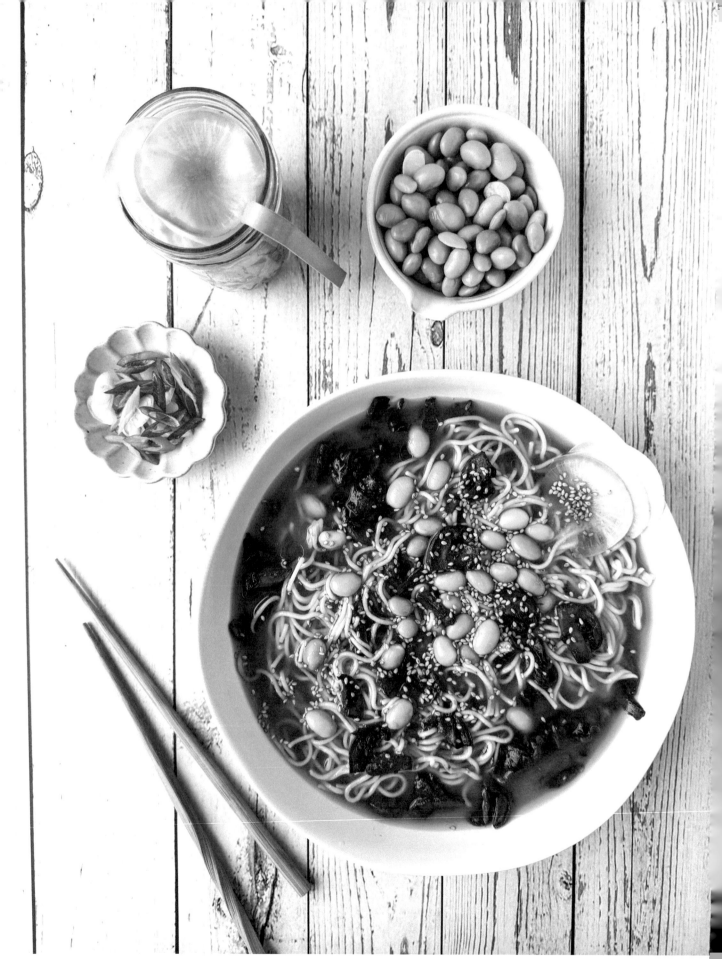

Garlic Miso Mushrooms

Makes about 4 servings

Sautéed mushrooms meet garlic, tamari, and white miso for a deep, savory umami flavor. Enjoy them as a flavorful side, stir them into ramen bowls, or add them to a nourish bowl for a delicious umami boost!

INGREDIENTS

- 16 ounces sliced cremini or white button mushrooms
- 1 tablespoon Tamari Lite
- 3 medium garlic cloves, minced
- 1 tablespoon white miso paste
- 2 tablespoons water

METHOD

1. Heat a large nonstick skillet over medium heat.
2. Once the skillet is hot, add the mushrooms and spread them into an even layer, stirring occasionally. Allow the mushrooms to release their liquid and start to brown, about 8 to 10 minutes.
3. Add the tamari and garlic and stir until evenly coated. Cook for 1 minute.
4. Turn the heat off. Whisk together the miso paste and water until smooth. Add to the mushrooms, scraping the flavor bits from the bottom of the pan.
5. Refrigerate leftovers in an airtight container for up to 4 days.

NUTRITIONAL INFORMATION (PER SERVING)

Per serving: Calories 37.1, Carbohydrate 5.4 g, Fiber 1.3 g, Total Sugars 2.3 g, Added Sugars 0 g, Fat 0.4 g, Saturated Fat 0.1 g, Protein 4.4 g, Sodium 306.3 mg, Iron 0.9 mg

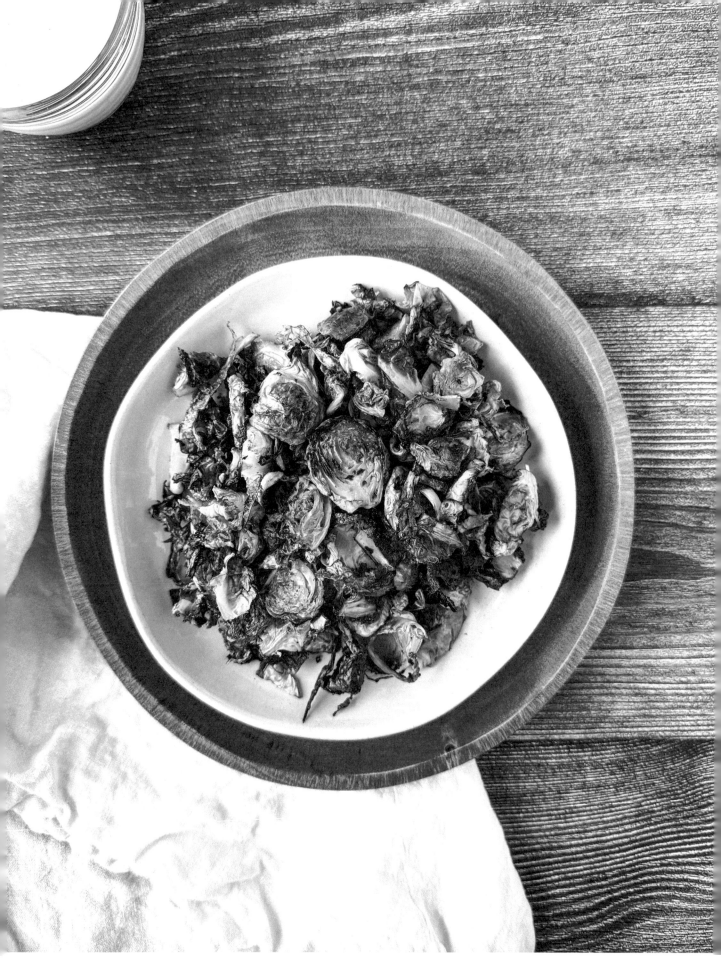

Balsamic Brussels Sprouts

Makes about 6 servings

Roasted until tender with crispy edges (Ted's favorite!), these Brussels sprouts are tossed in balsamic vinegar and a hint of pure maple syrup for a perfect balance of sweet and tangy. Enjoy them as a side dish or add them to roasted potatoes, salads, pasta, or nourish bowls!

INGREDIENTS

- 2 pounds brussels sprouts, stems removed and quartered lengthwise
- 2 tablespoons Tamari Lite
- 1 teaspoon garlic powder
- ¼ teaspoon freshly ground black pepper
- 2 tablespoons aged balsamic vinegar
- 2 teaspoons pure maple syrup

METHOD

1. Preheat oven to 425°F. Line a rimmed baking sheet with parchment paper.
2. Put the brussels sprouts in a medium bowl. Be sure to cut each brussels sprout into similar sizes to ensure even cooking. Add the tamari, garlic powder, and black pepper. Stir until evenly coated. Add to the lined baking sheet in a single layer.
3. Roast on the middle oven rack for about 18 minutes or until golden and tender. Stir halfway through cooking time.
4. Transfer to a serving bowl and drizzle with balsamic vinegar and maple syrup. Toss until evenly coated. Season with salt and pepper, if desired.
5. Refrigerate leftovers in an airtight container for up to 4 days.

NUTRITIONAL INFORMATION (PER SERVING)

Per serving: Calories 85.5, Carbohydrate 18 g, Fiber 5.8 g, Total Sugars 6.6 g, Added Sugars 1.3 g, Fat 0.5 g, Saturated Fat 0.1 g, Protein 5.5 g, Sodium 203.1 mg, Iron 2.6 mg

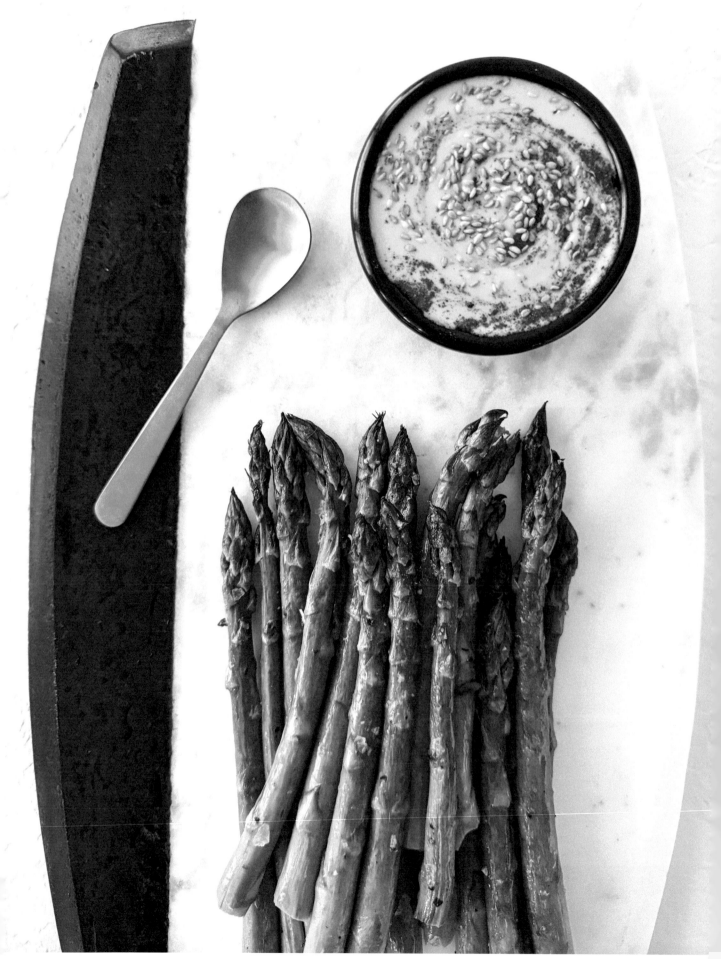

Roasted Asparagus

Makes about 4 servings

This recipe comes together quickly with just three ingredients. Fresh asparagus is tossed with a touch of extra-virgin olive oil and salt, then roasted until firm-tender. Enjoy as a side dish, or cut into bite-size pieces and add to pasta, salads, or nourish bowls.

INGREDIENTS

- 1 pound asparagus, woody ends trimmed
- 2 teaspoons extra-virgin olive oil
- ⅛ teaspoon salt

METHOD

1. Preheat oven to 425°F.
2. Place the asparagus on a rimmed baking sheet, drizzle with oil, and sprinkle with salt. Toss until evenly coated.
3. Roast on the middle rack for 6 to 10 minutes, or until lightly browned and tender when pierced with a fork. Thinner stems require less time than thicker stems.
4. Season with additional salt and freshly ground black pepper, if desired.
5. Refrigerate leftovers in an airtight container for up to 4 days.

NUTRITIONAL INFORMATION (PER SERVING)

Per serving: Calories 42.4, Carbohydrate 4.4 g, Fiber 2.4 g, Total Sugars 2.1 g, Added Sugars 0 g, Fat 2.4 g, Saturated Fat 0.4 g, Protein 2.5 g, Sodium 76 mg, Iron 2.4 mg

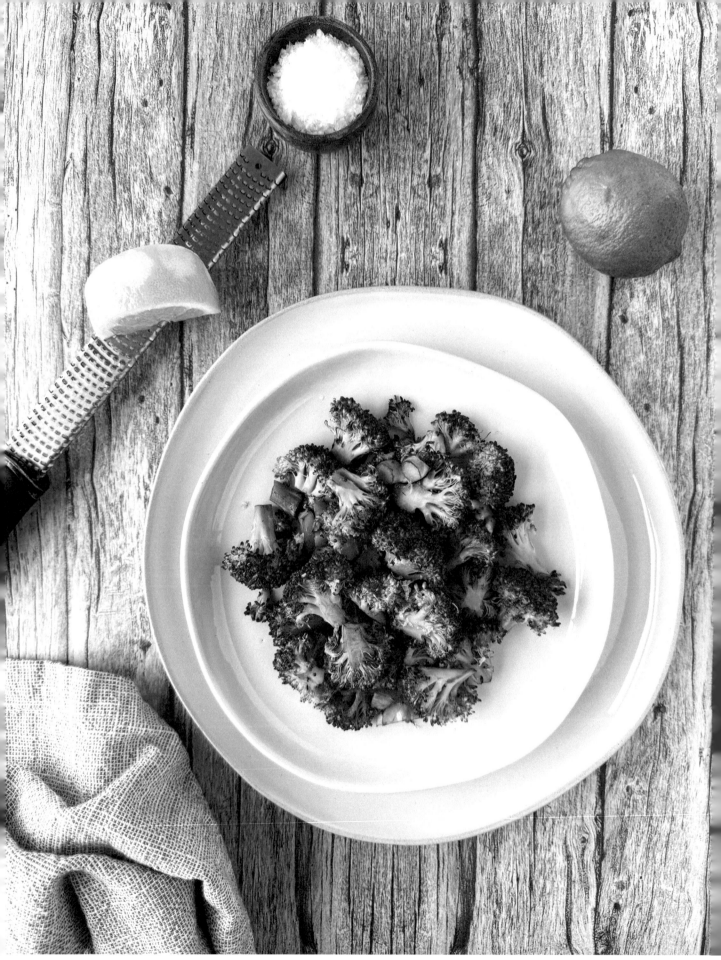

Sautéed Broccoli

Makes about 4 servings

Fresh broccoli is sautéed and tossed with fresh citrus juice and zest for a bright, refreshing flavor. It pairs wonderfully with pesto pasta and beans, nourish bowls, or as a simple side dish.

INGREDIENTS

- 1 large broccoli crown, cut into small bite-size pieces
- 2 tablespoons water
- 1 tablespoon fresh lemon or lime juice
- ⅛ teaspoon lemon or lime zest
- ⅛ teaspoon salt

METHOD

1. Heat a large skillet over medium-high heat. Add the broccoli and water. Cover and steam for 3 minutes.
2. Remove lid and continue to cook for another 2 to 3 minutes, or until crisp-tender and starting to turn golden brown on some sides.
3. Stir in the lemon or lime juice, zest, and salt.
4. Refrigerate leftovers in an airtight container for up to 4 days.

Flavor Tip:
Use lemon when pairing with Mediterranean and American dishes. Use lime when pairing with Latin and Asian dishes.

NUTRITIONAL INFORMATION (PER SERVING)

Per serving: Calories 52.5, Carbohydrate 10.3 g, Fiber 4 g, Total Sugars 2.7 g, Added Sugars 0 g, Fat 0.6 g, Saturated Fat 0.2 g, Protein 4.3 g, Sodium 124.2 mg, Iron 1.1 mg

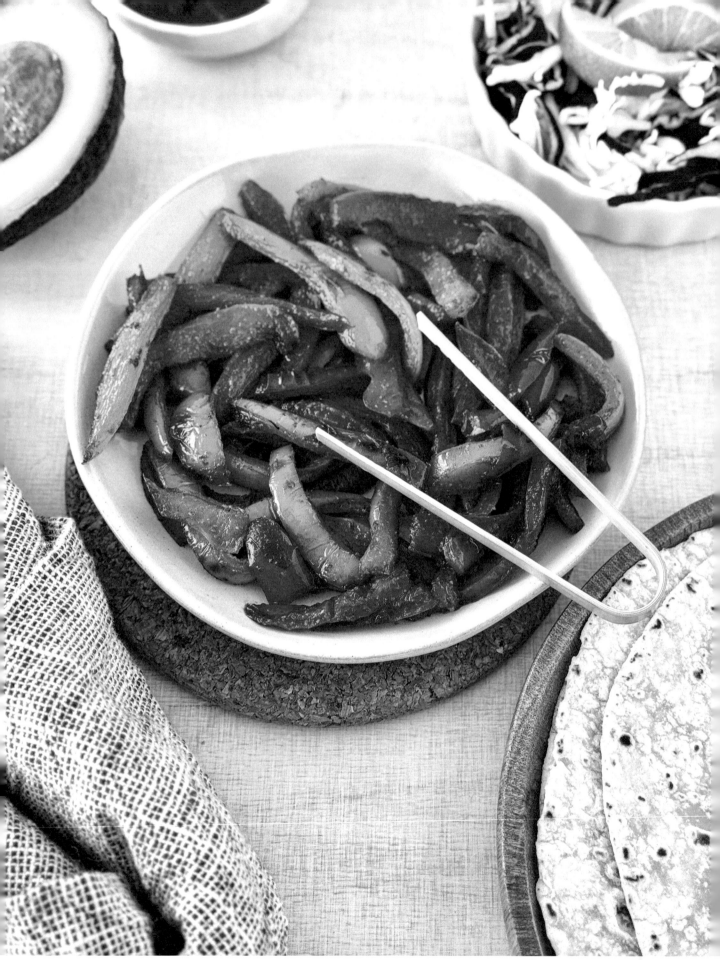

Sautéed Bell Peppers

Makes about 4 servings

Sliced and seasoned bell peppers are sautéed until soft, sweet, and lightly caramelized. They make a tasty topper for tacos, burrito bowls, Mediterranean salads, and hummus wraps.

INGREDIENTS

- 2 medium bell peppers (red, yellow, or orange), cut into ¼-inch slices
- 2 teaspoons extra-virgin olive oil
- ½ teaspoon garlic powder
- ¼ teaspoon salt
- ⅛ teaspoon smoked paprika

METHOD

1. Heat the oil in a large nonstick skillet over medium heat.
2. Add the sliced bell peppers to the skillet. Sprinkle with the garlic powder, salt, and smoked paprika. Stir until evenly coated.
3. Sauté the bell peppers, stirring occasionally, until soft, sweet, and lightly caramelized, about 10 to 12 minutes. Lower the heat if needed to prevent burning, and deglaze the skillet with a splash of water as needed.
4. Refrigerate leftovers in an airtight container for up to 4 days.

NUTRITIONAL INFORMATION (PER SERVING)

Per serving: Calories 36.7, Carbohydrate 3.9 g, Fiber 1.3 g, Total Sugars 2.5 g, Added Sugars 0 g, Fat 2.4 g, Saturated Fat 0.3 g, Protein 0.7 g, Sodium 150 mg, Iron 0.3 mg

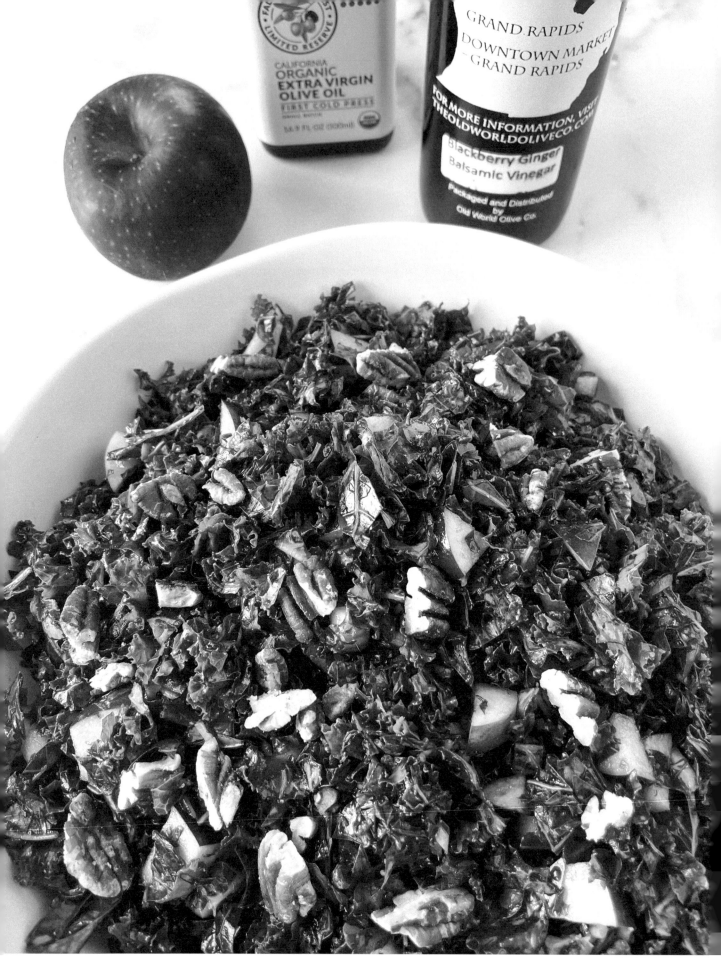

Massaged Kale Salad with Apples

Makes about 4 servings

This salad combines crisp apples, crunchy nuts, and a splash of aged balsamic vinegar. Massaging the kale softens its texture, reduces bitterness, and aids digestion. Enjoy as a side or as a main dish with farro or your favorite protein.

INGREDIENTS

- 1 (16-ounce) bunch curly kale, stems removed
- 1 tablespoon extra-virgin olive oil
- ⅛ teaspoon salt
- 1 tablespoon aged balsamic vinegar
- 1 teaspoon pure maple syrup
- 1 medium apple, cored and diced
- ¼ cup chopped toasted pecans

VARIATIONS

- Instead of apples, use dried unsweetened cranberries or cherries.
- Instead of pecans, use toasted walnuts or sliced almonds.
- Try a fruit-infused balsamic like pomegranate, fig, or blackberry.
- Add thinly sliced red onion.

METHOD

1. Chop the kale into small, bite-size pieces.
2. In a medium bowl, combine the chopped kale, oil, and a pinch of salt. Massage with your hands for about 2 minutes until softened and reduced by half.
3. Drizzle with the balsamic and maple syrup and toss until well combined. Season with additional salt and black pepper, if desired.
4. Stir in the apples and nuts. Best enjoyed immediately.

NUTRITIONAL INFORMATION (PER SERVING)

Per serving: Calories 153.3, Carbohydrate 15.1 g, Fiber 6.4 g, Total Sugars 8.6 g, Added Sugars 1 g, Fat 10.2 g, Saturated Fat 1.1 g, Protein 4.1 g, Sodium 135.8 mg, Iron 2.2 mg

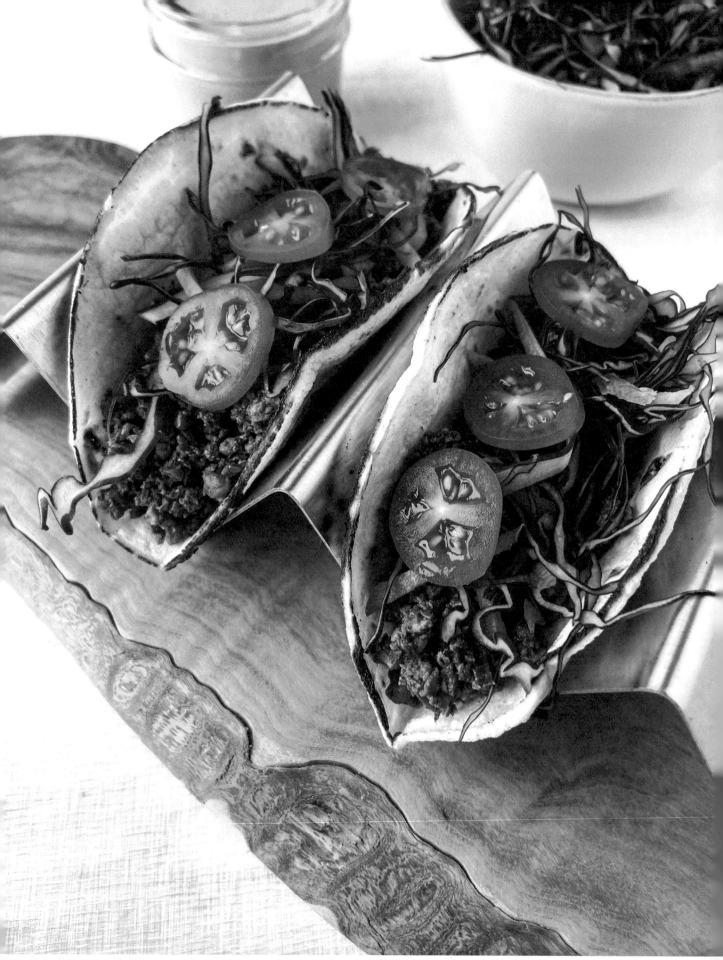

Mushroom Walnut Taco Filling

Makes about 4 servings

This is one of my most requested recipes from clients. Add this savory mixture to tacos, burritos, or enchiladas. Serve with your favorite toppings like crunchy cabbage slaw, tomatoes, and Cilantro Lime Crema (page 77) or Cashew Queso (page 75).

INGREDIENTS

- 16 ounces cremini or white button mushrooms, sliced
- 1 cup raw walnut pieces
- ¼ cup water
- 1 tablespoon tomato paste
- 1 tablespoon reduced-sodium tamari
- 1 tablespoon chili powder
- 1 tablespoon ground cumin
- ½ teaspoon smoked paprika
- 2 teaspoons extra-virgin olive oil
- ½ cup diced onion
- 4 medium garlic cloves, minced
- 1 tablespoon fresh lime juice

METHOD

1. If sliced mushrooms are unavailable, you can use whole mushrooms. Remove dirt with a damp paper towel. Cut in half for small mushrooms, and quarters for large.
2. Put the mushrooms in the food processor using the S-blade. Pulse until they have a ground meatlike texture, scraping down the sides of the food processor as needed. Empty into a large bowl.
3. Put the walnuts in the food processor and pulse into a fine crumble. Add to the bowl with mushrooms and stir until well combined.
4. In a small bowl, whisk together the water, tomato paste, and tamari until smooth.
5. In a small bowl, mix together the chili powder, cumin, and smoked paprika.
6. Heat the oil in a large nonstick skillet over medium heat. Once hot, add the onions and garlic, sautéing until the onions are translucent, about 3 minutes.
7. Add the dry spice mixture to the skillet and cook until aromatic, about 1 minute.
8. Add the mushroom and walnut mixture to the skillet along with the tomato paste and water mixture. Mix everything together until well combined. Cook the mixture for 8 to 10 minutes or until the liquid has absorbed, stirring occasionally. Continue cooking for another 4 minutes or until the mixture is dry and starts to brown, stirring to avoid burning.
9. Stir in the lime juice and taste. Season with salt and pepper, if desired.

NUTRITIONAL INFORMATION (PER SERVING)

Per serving: Calories 179, Carbohydrate 9.3 g, Fiber 3.1 g, Total Sugars 3.3 g, Added Sugars 0 g, Fat 14.9 g, Saturated Fat 1.5 g, Protein 6.4 g, Sodium 163.9 mg, Iron 2.1 mg

PLANT PROTEINS

Legumes

Plant proteins are often an overlooked and underutilized part of the diet. They are fiber-rich, lower in calories, and free of unhealthy saturated fats compared to many animal protein sources.

Incorporating more plant proteins can help support long-term health and longevity. Some well-known legumes include beans, chickpeas, lentils, and soybeans—all of which can be sautéed, roasted, mashed, or puréed to create delicious and nutritious meals.

The following recipes use canned beans, chickpeas, and lentils for convenience—perfect for quick, nourishing meals. When choosing canned options, look for non-BPA cans and avoid additives or oil for the cleanest ingredients.

If time allows, cooking dry legumes from scratch is a more budget-friendly and customizable option. It gives you full control over ingredients, reduces sodium, and enhances flavor and texture. Plus, cooking a big batch and freezing portions makes meal prep even easier. Whether you go with canned or dried, legumes are a versatile, nutrient-packed addition to any plant-based meal!

- Easy Beans
- Roasted Chickpeas
- Cranberry Walnut Chickpea Salad
- Curried Chickpea Salad
- Tofu: Different Types + How to Prepare
- Tofu Cubes: 4 Ways (oven + air fryer method)
  - Simple Tofu Cubes
  - Balsamic Herb Tofu Cubes
  - Garlic Paprika Tofu Cubes
  - Chili Lime Tofu Cubes
- Saucy Asian Tofu Cubes
- Mediterranean Tofu Feta
- Tofu Taco Meat
- Unk's Tofu Larb Lettuce Wraps

- Tofu Ricotta
- Shelled Edamame
- Easy Lentil Marinara
- Herby Lentils with Olives
- Tempeh: Different Types + How to Prepare
  - Buffalo Tempeh Crumbles
  - Asian Tempeh Cubes

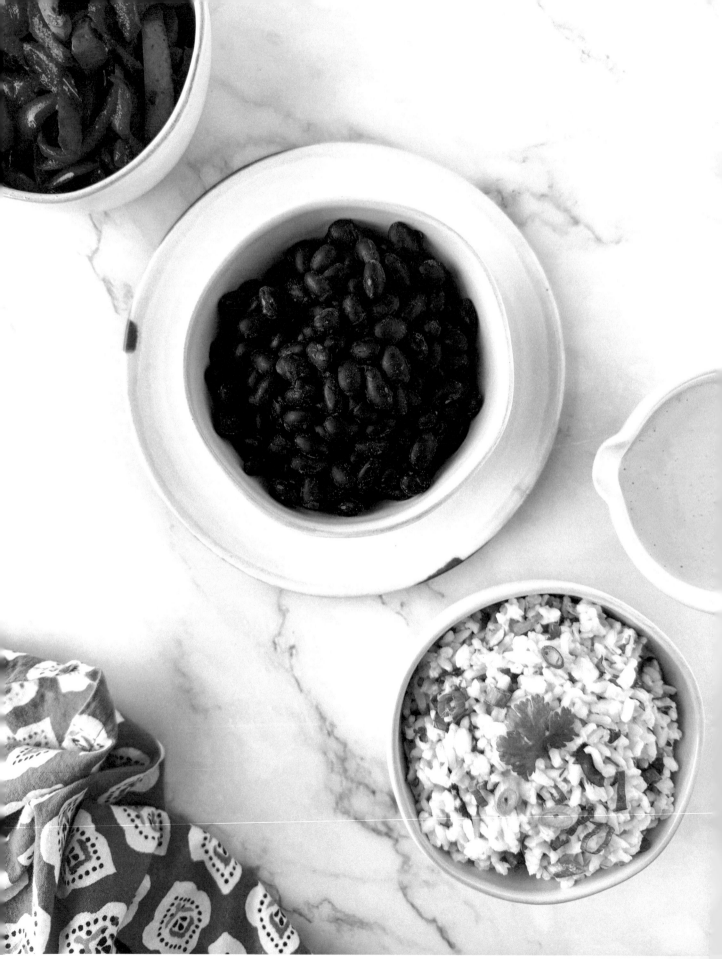

Easy Beans

Makes about 4 servings

Let's face it. Beans straight out of the can often lack flavor and taste tinny—not exactly appetizing. When you don't have time to cook dry beans, try this quick and easy method to transform those bland beans into a flavorful delight! The secret? Heat the beans with a bit of salt, then toss them with some acid, like vinegar. Make a batch or two on your weekly meal prep day for a quick protein source that can be added to salads, bowls, and wraps.

INGREDIENTS

- 1 (15-ounce) can of beans, chickpeas, or lentils, rinsed and drained, *see note**
- ¼ teaspoon salt, or to taste
- 1 teaspoon red or white wine vinegar

*Note:
This recipe works well with red kidney beans, black beans, cannellini beans, and pinto beans.

METHOD

1. Add the beans and salt to a microwave-safe bowl and stir until combined. Cover and microwave on high until hot, about 1 ½ minutes.
2. While the beans are still hot, stir in the vinegar and allow to cool.
3. Refrigerate leftovers in an airtight container for 4 days.

Flavor Tip:
Stir in a teaspoon of your favorite dried spices in place of the salt before heating.

NUTRITIONAL INFORMATION (PER SERVING)

Per serving: Calories 82, Carbohydrate 13.1 g, Fiber 3.3 g, Total Sugars 0 g, Added Sugars 0 g, Fat 1.6 g, Saturated Fat 0 g, Protein 4.1 g, Sodium 157.65 mg, Iron 1.3 mg

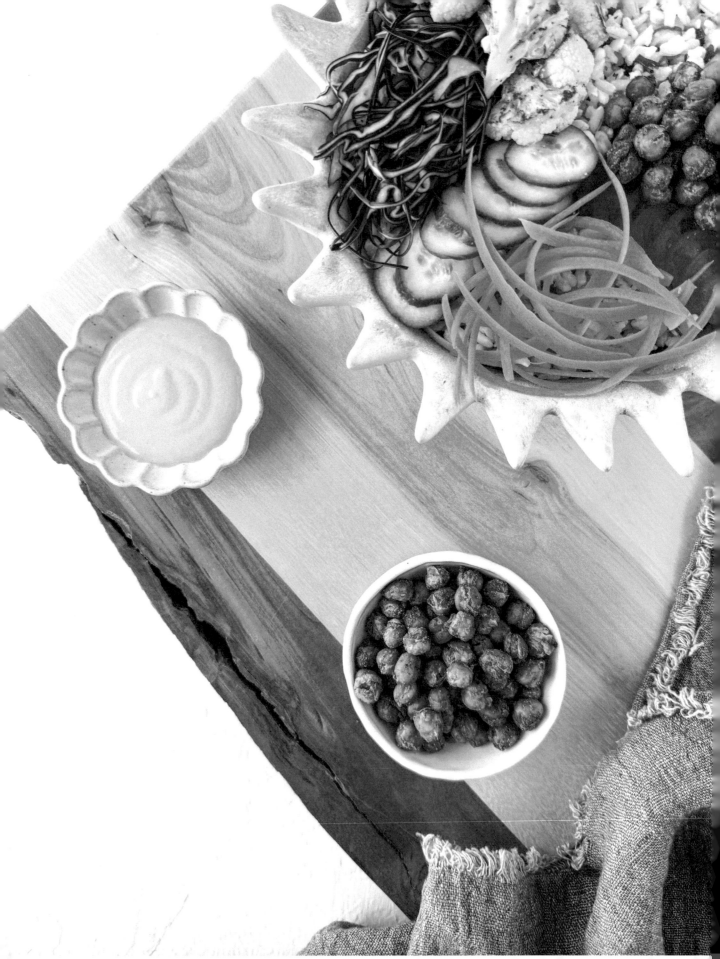

Roasted Chickpeas

Makes about 4 servings

Crispy, seasoned, and packed with protein, roasted chickpeas are perfect for salads, nourish bowls, soup toppers, or as a satisfying snack!

INGREDIENTS

- 1 (15-ounce) can chickpeas, rinsed and drained
- ½ teaspoon ground paprika
- ½ teaspoon ground cumin
- ½ teaspoon garlic powder
- ½ teaspoon salt
- ½ teaspoon arrowroot starch (or cornstarch)
- ¼ teaspoon onion powder
- ¼ teaspoon smoked paprika
- ⅛ teaspoon freshly ground black pepper
- 2 teaspoons extra-virgin olive oil

METHOD

1. Preheat oven to 400°F. Line a large rimmed baking sheet with parchment paper.
2. Place the drained chickpeas on a kitchen towel to remove excess water.
3. In a medium bowl, combine the spices. Add the oil and chickpeas and gently mix until evenly coated.
4. Transfer the seasoned chickpeas to the baking sheet and gently spread into a single layer. Bake for 20 minutes on the middle oven rack. Stir the beans and return to the oven for 15 more minutes or until golden and crispy. (For extra-crispy results: Turn the oven off and leave the chickpeas in the oven for 8 to 10 minutes.)
5. For best results, enjoy immediately.
6. Once cooled, store leftovers in an airtight container at room temperature for 2 to 3 days.

NUTRITIONAL INFORMATION (PER SERVING)

Per serving: Calories 172.6, Carbohydrate 25.0 g, Fiber 7.0 g, Total Sugars 4.3 g, Added Sugars 0 g, Fat 5.3 g, Saturated Fat 0.6 g, Protein 7.7 g, Sodium 521.1 mg, Iron 1.3 mg

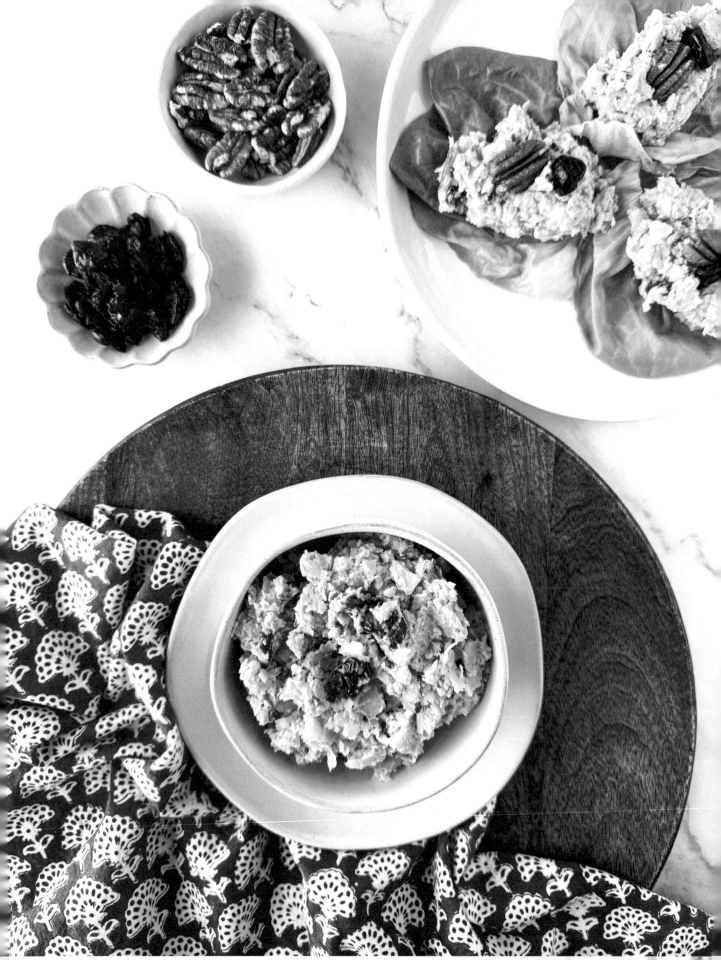

Cranberry Walnut Chickpea Salad

Makes about 8 servings

Chickpeas are combined with vegan mayo, crunchy celery, red onion, dried cranberries, and toasted nuts. Add a scoop of Cranberry Walnut Chickpea Salad to a bed of greens with a healthy drizzle of Balsamic Walnut Dressing (page 51), or on toasted sourdough bread for a delicious open-faced sandwich.

INGREDIENTS

- 2 (15-ounce) cans chickpeas, drained and rinsed
- 2 tablespoons vegan mayonnaise, *see note**
- 2 teaspoons Dijon mustard
- ½ teaspoon salt
- 2 medium celery ribs, diced
- 2 tablespoons minced red onion
- ⅓ cup chopped toasted walnuts (or pecans)
- ⅓ cup dried cranberries, unsweetened

METHOD

1. In a food processor with the S-blade, combine the chickpeas, mayonnaise, Dijon, and salt. Process until mostly smooth with a few chunks, scraping the sides down as needed. Transfer to a medium bowl. Alternatively, you can use a potato masher.
2. Stir in the celery, red onion, walnuts, and cranberries until well combined.
3. Refrigerate leftovers in an airtight container for up to 5 days.

*Note:
Use 2 tablespoons of
Cashew Cream
(page 43) in place of
vegan mayonnaise.

NUTRITIONAL INFORMATION (PER SERVING)

Per serving: Calories 193.3, Carbohydrate 26.5 g, Fiber 7.6 g, Total Sugars 5 g, Added Sugars 0 g, Fat 6.8 g, Saturated Fat 0.6 g, Protein 8.4 g, Sodium 433.9 mg, Iron 1.2 mg

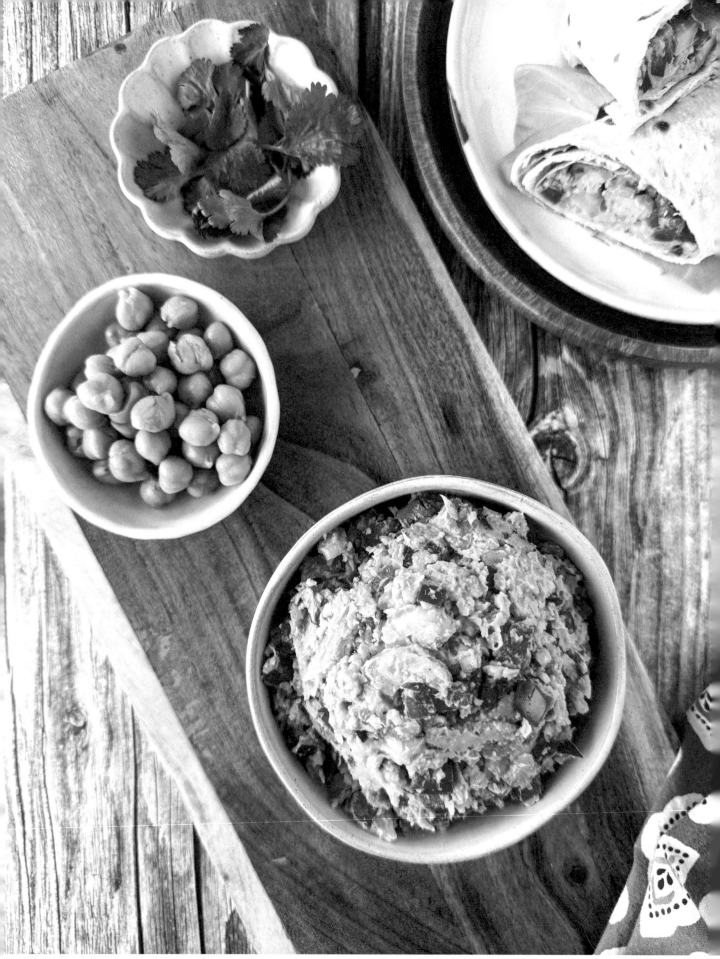

Curried Chickpea Salad

Makes about 8 servings

Chickpeas are combined with Indian spices and a variety of fresh vegetables for a flavorful and nutritious dish. Serve with toasted whole-grain naan or in crispy lettuce cups for a quick grab-and-go meal!

INGREDIENTS

- 2 (15-ounce) can chickpeas, drained and rinsed
- 2 tablespoons vegan mayonnaise, *see note**
- 2 teaspoons Dijon mustard
- 1 teaspoon curry powder
- ½ teaspoon turmeric powder
- ½ teaspoon salt
- 1 medium red bell pepper, finely diced
- 2 medium celery ribs, finely diced
- 2 tablespoons minced red onion
- ½ cup firmly packed fresh cilantro leaves, chopped

METHOD

1. In a food processor fitted with an S-blade, combine the chickpeas, mayonnaise, Dijon, curry powder, turmeric, and salt. Process until mostly smooth with a few chunks, scraping down the sides as needed. Transfer to a medium bowl. (For a chunkier texture, you can also mash by hand using a potato masher)

2. Stir in the bell pepper, celery, red onion, and cilantro until well combined.

3. Refrigerate leftovers in an airtight container for up to 5 days.

*Note:
Use 2 tablespoons of Cashew Cream (page 43) in place of vegan mayonnaise.

NUTRITIONAL INFORMATION (PER SERVING)

Per serving: Calories 163.8, Carbohydrate 26.1 g, Fiber 7.6 g, Total Sugars 5.3 g, Added Sugars 0 g, Fat 3.7 g, Saturated Fat 0.3 g, Protein 7.9 g, Sodium 434.3 mg, Iron 1.3 mg

Tofu: Different Types + How to Prepare

Tofu, derived from soy milk, is a wonderfully adaptable protein that acts like a sponge, ready to soak up any seasonings and marinades you add. Available in various textures like silken, regular, firm, extra-firm, and super-firm, tofu can be used in everything from smoothies and soups to stir-fries and desserts. It's low in calories but high in protein, vitamins, and essential minerals like calcium and iron. If you haven't enjoyed tofu in the past, I encourage you to give it another try. My family and clients are huge fans, and my simple tips and tricks might make you a fan, too!

Types of Tofu: Choose organic tofu whenever possible, as soy is commonly genetically modified in the U.S. In this cookbook, we'll be using super-firm, extra-firm, and firm tofu blocks found in the refrigerated section of your market. Avoid silken tofu varieties for these recipes, as they are too soft and delicate.

Super-Firm

- Similar texture to meat
- No pressing required, saving time
- Can be crumbled, cut, or torn into different shapes

Extra-Firm

- Similar texture to scrambled eggs
- Press to remove excess water
- Can be crumbled, cut, or torn into different shapes

Firm

- Similar texture to ricotta cheese
- Wrap with a paper towel and quickly press with your hands
- Can be crumbled or mashed into a smooth paste

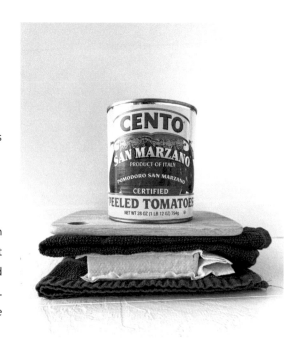

Tofu: How to Press

For best results with extra-firm tofu, pressing is required. Drain and rinse the tofu, then wrap it in a clean dish towel. Set a flat baking sheet or cutting board on top of the tofu block, and add a heavy cookbook or a large tomato can for additional weight. Let it press for 15 to 30 minutes. This process will allow the tofu to absorb more flavor from seasonings and marinades.

Tofu: How to Cut

Tofu can be cut into many different shapes, like planks, strips, triangles, and cubes. Our versatile go-to method is cubed tofu, which can be added to bowls, wraps, and salads.

1. Place the tofu block on its side on a cutting board. Cut lengthwise into about ¾-inch planks. You will end up with either two or three pieces, depending on the size of the block.
2. Evenly stack the planks from top to bottom and cut each plank vertically into about ¾-inch strips.
3. Rotate the strips 90 degrees, then cut them into evenly sized cubes.

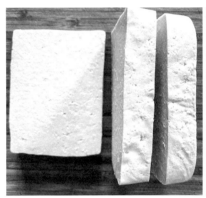 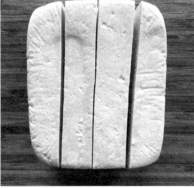 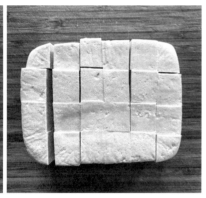

Tips: Tofu planks are the perfect shape for grilling or pan-frying, then tossing with your favorite sauce. Serve as a sandwich or burger, or on a plate with roasted veggies.

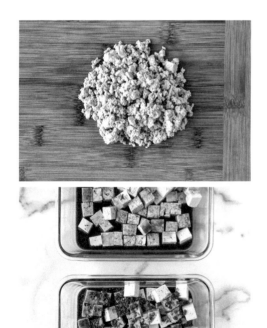

Tofu: How to Crumble

Use your hands or a potato masher to crumble into small pieces.

Tofu: How to Marinate

Add your marinade ingredients to a medium bowl or a large storage container and whisk until combined. Add the tofu to the marinade and gently toss until evenly coated. Cover and refrigerate for a minimum of 15 minutes, or overnight for best results.

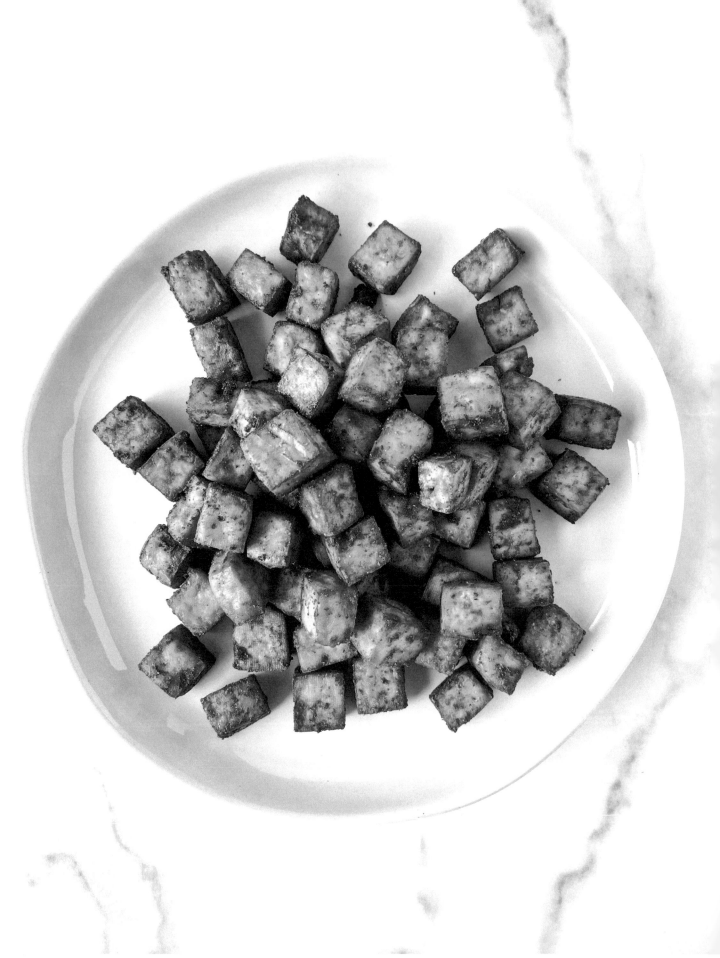

Tofu Cubes: 4 Ways

Each recipe makes about 4 servings

Cubed tofu with four flavorful marinades, cooked two different ways! Say goodbye to bland tofu with these delicious variations: Simple, Garlic Paprika, Balsamic Herb, and Chili Lime. Choose a marinade and cooking method below and make a batch on your meal prep day. Enjoy roasted tofu cubes in salads, nourish bowls, or handhelds with your favorite sauce or dressing.

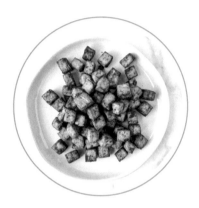

SIMPLE TOFU CUBES

- 1 (16-ounce) block super-firm tofu, *see note**
- 2 tablespoons reduced-sodium tamari
- 1 teaspoon arrowroot starch (or cornstarch)

NUTRITIONAL INFORMATION (PER SERVING)

Per Serving: Calories 170.3, Carbohydrate 3.7 g, Fiber 2.6 g, Total Sugars 0.2 g, Added Sugars 0 g, Fat 8.7 g, Saturated Fat 1.9 g, Protein 18.4 g, Sodium 362.7 mg, Iron 2.5 mg

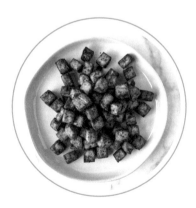

GARLIC PAPRIKA TOFU CUBES

- 1 (16-ounce) block super-firm tofu, *see note**
- 2 tablespoons reduced-sodium tamari
- 1 teaspoon garlic powder
- 1 teaspoon paprika
- 1 teaspoon arrowroot starch (or cornstarch)
- ¼ teaspoon onion powder

NUTRITIONAL INFORMATION (PER SERVING)

Per Serving: Calories 174.5, Carbohydrate 4.6 g, Fiber 2.9 g, Total Sugars 0.2 g, Added Sugars 0 g, Fat 8.8 g, Saturated Fat 1.9 g, Protein 18.6 g, Sodium 363.7 mg, Iron 2.6 mg

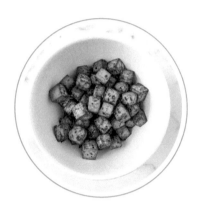

BALSAMIC HERB TOFU CUBES

- 1 (16-ounce) block super-firm tofu, *see note**
- 1 tablespoon aged balsamic vinegar
- 1 tablespoon reduced-sodium tamari
- 1 tablespoon Dijon mustard
- 1 teaspoon dried oregano
- 1 teaspoon arrowroot starch (or cornstarch)
- ½ teaspoon garlic powder
- ½ teaspoon pure maple syrup

NUTRITIONAL INFORMATION (PER SERVING)

Calories 182.5, Carbohydrate 6.3 g, Fiber 2.8 g, Total Sugars 2.1 g, Added Sugars 0.5 g, Fat 9 g, Saturated Fat 1.9 g, Protein 18.2 g, Sodium 279.1 mg, Iron 2.7 mg

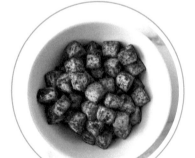

CHILI LIME TOFU CUBES

- 1 (16-ounce) block super-firm tofu, *see note**
- 1 tablespoon lime juice
- 1 tablespoon reduced-sodium tamari
- 2 teaspoons chili powder
- 1 teaspoon garlic powder
- 1 teaspoon arrowroot starch (or cornstarch)
- ½ teaspoon cumin powder
- ½ teaspoon salt (optional)

NUTRITIONAL INFORMATION (PER SERVING)

Calories 175.4, Carbohydrate 5 g, Fiber 3.1 g, Total Sugars 0.3 g, Added Sugars 0 g, Fat 9 g, Saturated Fat 1.9 g, Protein 18.3 g, Sodium 521.6 mg, Iron 2.8 mg

OVEN METHOD

Prepare the tofu: Drain and rinse the tofu. Pat it dry with paper towels. Cut the tofu into ½- to ¾-inch cubes.

Preheat oven to 400°F. Line a large rimmed baking sheet with parchment paper.

Marinate: In a medium container with a leak-proof lid, combine the marinade ingredients and whisk together until well combined. Add the tofu cubes to the marinade and cover with an airtight lid, gently shaking until the tofu is evenly coated. Marinate for a minimum of 15 minutes or overnight in the refrigerator.

Roast: Remove the tofu from the marinade with a slotted spoon and add to the baking sheet in a single layer, making sure not to crowd the cubes. Roast on the middle rack for 25 to 30 minutes or until golden brown on the edges. Discard excess marinade or save for another recipe.

Leftovers: Allow the tofu to cool before storing in the refrigerator in an airtight container for 4 to 5 days.

AIR FRYER METHOD

Prepare the tofu: Drain and rinse the tofu. Pat it dry with paper towels. Cut the tofu into ½-inch to ¾-inch cubes.

Marinate: In a medium container with a leak-proof lid, combine the marinade ingredients and whisk together until well combined. Add the tofu cubes to the marinade and cover with an airtight lid, gently shaking until the tofu is evenly coated. Marinate for a minimum of 15 minutes or overnight in the refrigerator.

Cook: Remove the tofu from the marinade with a slotted spoon and add to the air fryer basket. Cook at 400°F for about 15 minutes or until crispy and golden. Shake the basket every 5 minutes to ensure even cooking. Discard excess marinade or save for another recipe.

Leftovers: Allow the tofu to cool before storing in the refrigerator in an airtight container for 4 to 5 days.

*Note:
If super-firm tofu is unavailable, use extra-firm tofu that has been pressed. Using extra-firm tofu will change the nutritional analysis.

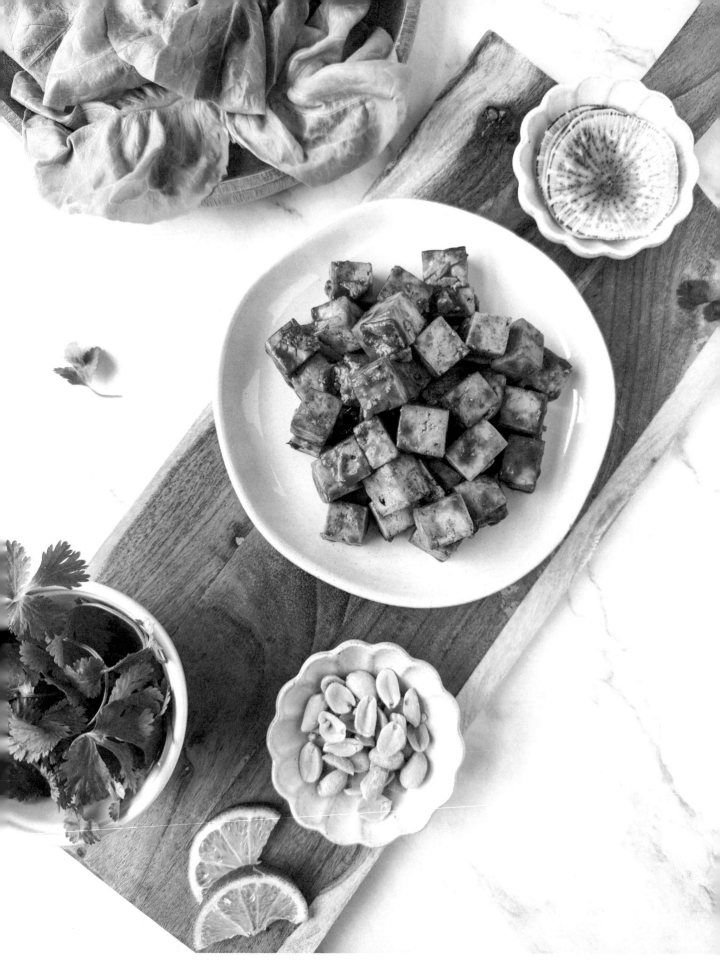

Sweet Sriracha Tofu Cubes

Makes about 4 servings

Tofu cubes are combined with a tasty marinade, then sautéed in a skillet. Try pairing these saucy cubes with crispy lettuce cups or with steamed broccoli and soba noodles, sprinkled with toasted sesame seeds and sliced green onions

INGREDIENTS

- 1 (16-ounce) block super-firm tofu*
- 3 tablespoons reduced-sodium tamari
- 2 tablespoons fresh lime juice
- 1 tablespoon + 1 teaspoon pure maple syrup
- 1 tablespoon sriracha
- 2 teaspoons arrowroot starch (or cornstarch)
- 1 teaspoon toasted sesame oil

*Note:
If super-firm tofu is unavailable, use extra-firm tofu that has been pressed. Using extra-firm tofu will change the nutritional analysis.

METHOD

1. Prepare the tofu: Drain and rinse the tofu. Pat it dry with paper towels. Cut the tofu into ½-inch to ¾-inch cubes.

2. Marinate: In a medium container with a leak-proof lid, combine the marinade ingredients and whisk together until well combined. Add the tofu cubes to the marinade and cover with an airtight lid, gently shaking until the tofu is evenly coated. Marinate for a minimum of 15 minutes or overnight in the refrigerator.

3. Cook: Preheat a large nonstick skillet over medium heat. Using a slotted spoon, remove the tofu and place in the skillet. Save the remaining marinade. Sauté the tofu until golden brown on most sides, tossing every few minutes, about 6 minutes.

4. Turn the heat off and carefully add the remaining marinade, gently tossing until evenly coated and warmed through.

NUTRITIONAL INFORMATION (PER SERVING)

Calories 195.4, Carbohydrate 7.1 g, Fiber 2.8 g, Total Sugars 5.1 g, Added Sugars 4.6 g, Fat 9.9 g, Saturated Fat 2 g, Protein 19 g, Sodium 641.7 mg, Iron 2.7 mg

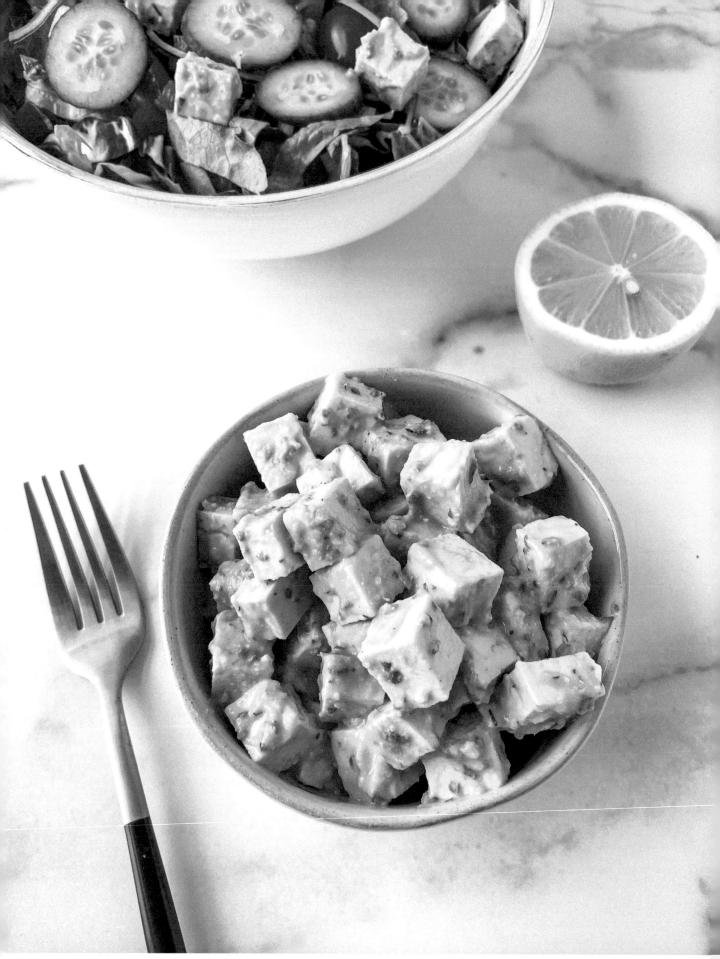

Mediterranean Tofu Feta

Makes about 6 servings

This marinated tofu is a client favorite, including the kiddos! It pairs perfectly with Greek salads, pita sandwiches, and chilled pasta salads loaded with veggies.

INGREDIENTS

- 2 tablespoons white miso paste
- 2 tablespoons fresh lemon juice
- 2 tablespoons water
- 2 tablespoons nutritional yeast
- 1 tablespoon dried oregano
- ½ teaspoon garlic powder
- ½ teaspoon salt
- 1 (16-ounce) block super-firm tofu*, cubed

METHOD

1. In a medium bowl, combine the miso paste, lemon juice, water, nutritional yeast, oregano, garlic powder, and salt, and whisk until combined. Gently stir in the tofu cubes until evenly coated. Allow to marinate in the refrigerator for a minimum of 30 minutes prior to serving or overnight for best results.
2. Serve cold or at room temperature.
3. Refrigerate leftovers in an airtight container for up to 7 days.

*Note:
If super-firm tofu is unavailable, use extra-firm tofu that has been pressed. Using extra-firm tofu will change the nutritional analysis.

NUTRITIONAL INFORMATION (PER SERVING)

Calories 126.3, Carbohydrate 4.2 g, Fiber 2.4 g, Total Sugars 0.2 g, Added Sugars 0 g, Fat 5.9 g, Saturated Fat 1.3 g, Protein 13.4 g, Sodium 445.3 mg, Iron 1.8 mg

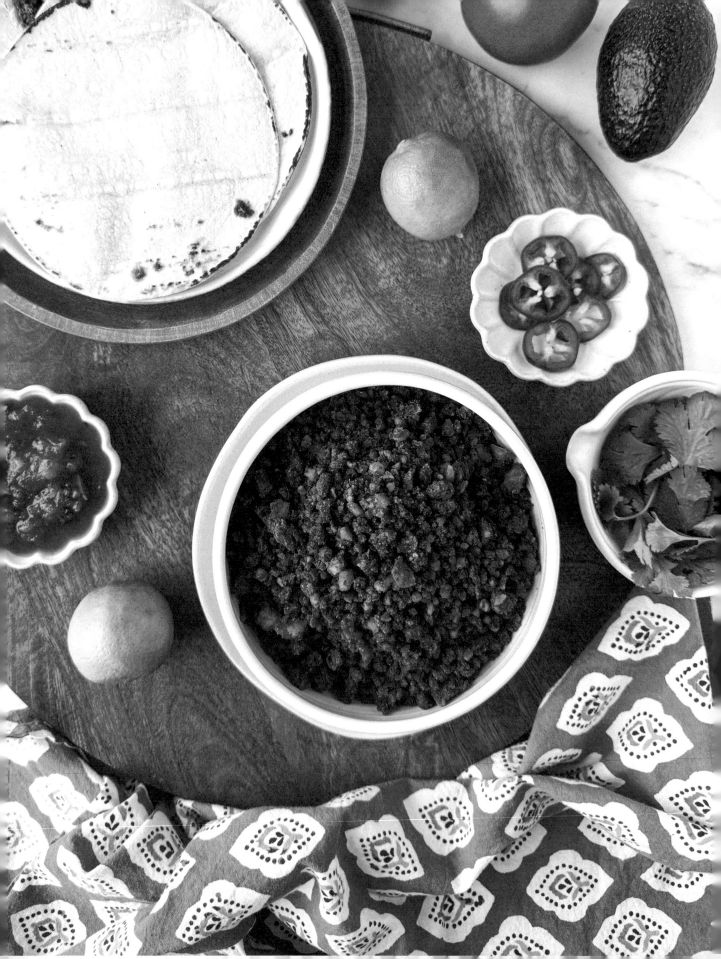

Tofu Taco Meat

Makes about 6 servings

Tofu taco meat is made with crumbled walnuts and tofu combined with a flavorful paste, then roasted until crispy and golden. Use this delicious filling for tacos, enchiladas, nachos, and burritos, or add it to your favorite chili in place of ground beef.

INGREDIENTS

- 2 tablespoons reduced-sodium tamari
- 2 tablespoons tomato paste
- 1 tablespoon nutritional yeast
- 1 tablespoon extra-virgin olive oil
- ½ tablespoon pure maple syrup
- 2 teaspoons chili powder
- ½ teaspoon garlic powder
- ½ teaspoon smoked paprika
- ¼ teaspoon cayenne pepper, or to taste
- 1 cup raw walnut pieces, small crumbles
- 1 (14-ounce) block extra-firm tofu, drained
- 1 tablespoon fresh lime juice

NUTRITIONAL INFORMATION (PER SERVING)

Calories 240.4, Carbohydrate 7.4 g, Fiber 2.5 g, Total Sugars 3 g, Added Sugars 1 g, Fat 19.8 g, Saturated Fat 2.3 g, Protein 13.3 g, Sodium 268.2 mg, Iron 3 mg

METHOD

1. Preheat oven to 350°F. Line a rimmed baking sheet with parchment paper.

2. In a medium bowl, combine the tamari, tomato paste, nutritional yeast, olive oil, maple syrup, chili powder, garlic powder, smoked paprika, and cayenne. Whisk into a paste.

3. Put the walnuts in a food processor with the S-blade. Pulse into small crumbles, similar to the size of a rice grain. Add to the spice mixture.

4. Give the tofu a quick squeeze between both palms to remove excess water. Add to the bowl with spices and walnuts. Mash the tofu with a potato masher or large fork. Stir everything together until well combined.

5. Transfer the mixture to the baking sheet and spread out evenly in a single layer across the tray. Bake in the oven on the middle rack for 35 to 45 minutes, or until golden and crispy on the edges. Stir every 15 minutes to ensure even cooking.

6. Squeeze half a lime over the tofu mixture and stir. Taste and season with salt, if desired.

7. Refrigerate leftovers in an airtight container for up to 5 days.

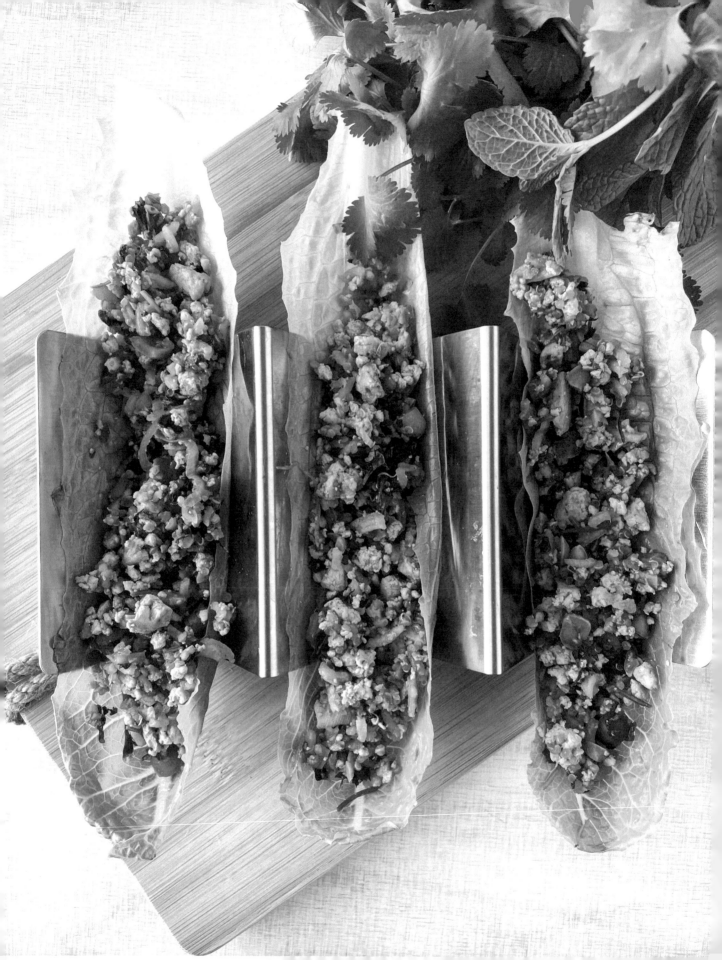

Unk's Tofu Larb Lettuce Wraps

This recipe is inspired by my uncle and aunt's personal chef from their time in Laos and has become a beloved favorite among clients and family! Packed with herby, umami-rich flavors and a delightful mix of textures, it's perfect served in crisp lettuce cups for a fresh and satisfying bite.

INGREDIENTS

- 1 cup cooked basmati brown rice*
- 1 tablespoon toasted sesame oil
- ½ cup finely diced white onion
- 1-inch piece jalapeño, seeds and ribs removed, minced
- 2 teaspoons minced fresh ginger
- 1 medium garlic clove, minced
- 1 (14-ounce) block of extra-firm tofu, crumbled
- ½ cup low-sodium vegetable broth

- 3 tablespoons reduced-sodium tamari
- 2 tablespoons fresh lime juice
- 1 tablespoon sriracha, more for garnish
- 2 cups fresh cilantro leaves, packed loosely, then chopped
- 2 cups fresh mint leaves, packed loosely, then chopped
- ½ cup chopped unsalted roasted peanuts

FOR SERVING (OPTIONAL)

- Crispy lettuce cups
- Avocado, cucumber, scallions, sriracha

*Note:
I often use ready-to-heat rice pouches to save time. Alternatively, you can cook ⅓ cup dry rice before you prep the other ingredients. Quinoa also works well in this recipe.

recipe continued onto next page...

Unk's Tofu Larb Lettuce Wraps, cont'd

METHOD

1. Heat the oil in a large skillet over medium heat. Add the onion, jalapeño, and a pinch of salt and cook until softened, about 3 minutes.
2. Stir in the ginger and garlic and cook until fragrant, about 1 minute.
3. Add the crumbled tofu and sauté for 6 to 8 minutes, or until the tofu starts to become golden.
4. In the meantime, make the sauce. In a small bowl, whisk together the broth, tamari, lime juice, and sriracha.
5. To the skillet, add the sauce, rice, cilantro, mint, and peanuts and stir until combined with the tofu mixture. Cook until the sauce reduces, about 3 minutes.
6. Serve warm or cold in lettuce leaves.
7. Refrigerate leftovers in an airtight container for up to 7 days.

Flavor Tip:
Marinate sliced
hot peppers in
tamari and use as
a spicy topper.

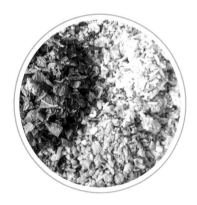

NUTRITIONAL INFORMATION
(PER SERVING)

Calories 247.3, Carbohydrate 20.1 g, Fiber 5.7 g,
Total Sugars 3.7 g, Added Sugars 0.2 g,
Fat 13.8 g, Saturated Fat 2.3 g, Protein 15.8 g,
Sodium 407.3 mg, Iron 6.7 mg

Plant Proteins: Legumes

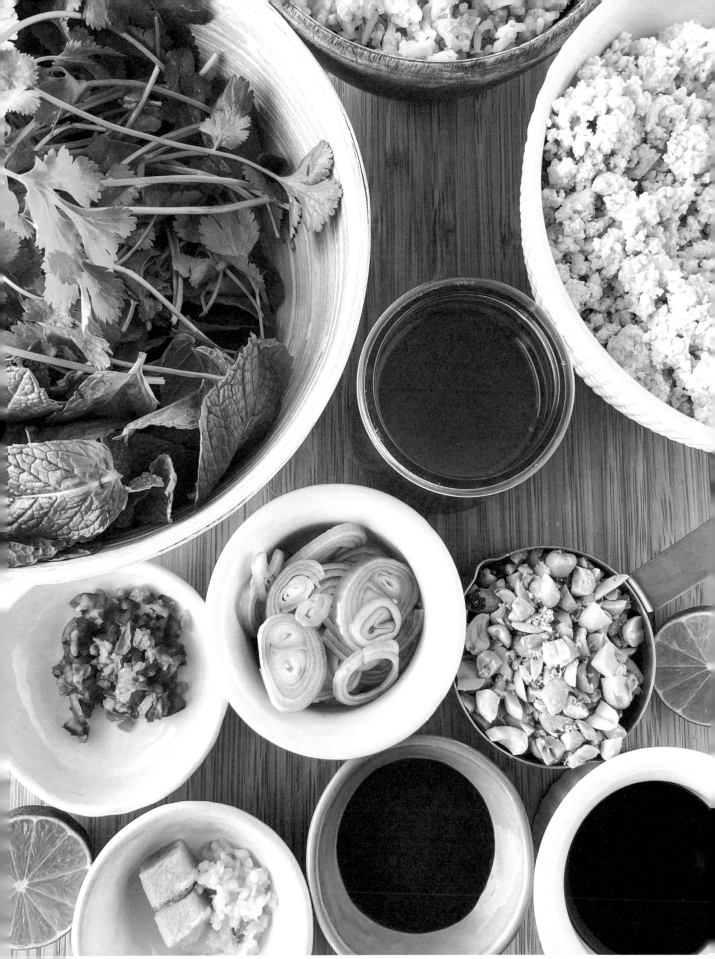

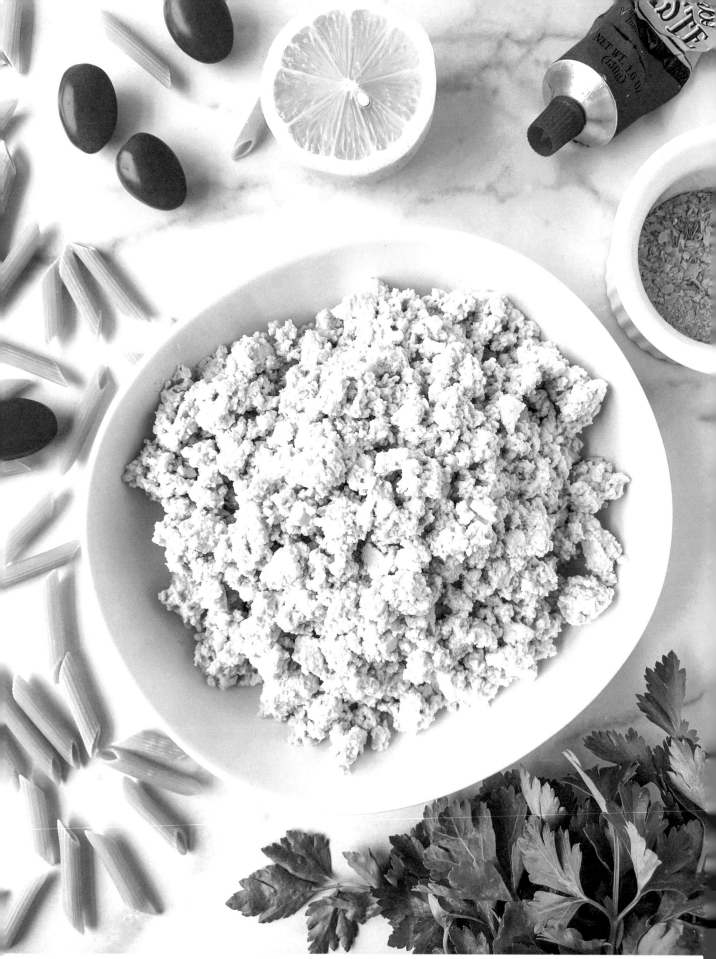

Tofu Ricotta

Makes about 6 servings

Layer this dairy-free ricotta in lasagna or warm pasta dishes, or add dollops on top of homemade pizza. For a quick lunch or snack, spread Tofu Ricotta on toasted sourdough bread and top with ripe tomatoes, fresh basil, and a drizzle of balsamic glaze.

INGREDIENTS

- 1 (14-ounce) block firm tofu, drained
- 2 tablespoons nutritional yeast
- 1 tablespoon fresh lemon juice
- 1 tablespoon white miso paste
- 2 medium garlic cloves, minced
- ½ teaspoon salt

VARIATIONS

1. Stir in 1 cup chopped fresh baby spinach.
2. Stir in 1 teaspoon each dried oregano and dried thyme.

METHOD

1. Wrap the drained tofu with a paper towel and gently squeeze the excess water with flat palms. Set aside.
2. In a medium bowl, combine the nutritional yeast, lemon juice, miso, garlic, and salt. Whisk until smooth.
3. Using your hands or a potato masher, crumble the block of tofu into the bowl. Stir until everything is well combined and the tofu is evenly coated, breaking up any larger pieces as needed.
4. Refrigerate leftovers in an airtight container for up to 3 days.

NUTRITIONAL INFORMATION (PER SERVING)

Per serving: Calories 81.5, Carbohydrate 4.2 g, Fiber 1.2 g, Total Sugars 0.6 g, Added Sugars 0 g, Fat 3.7 g, Saturated Fat 0.7 g, Protein 9.4 g, Sodium 328.9 mg, Iron 1.6 mg

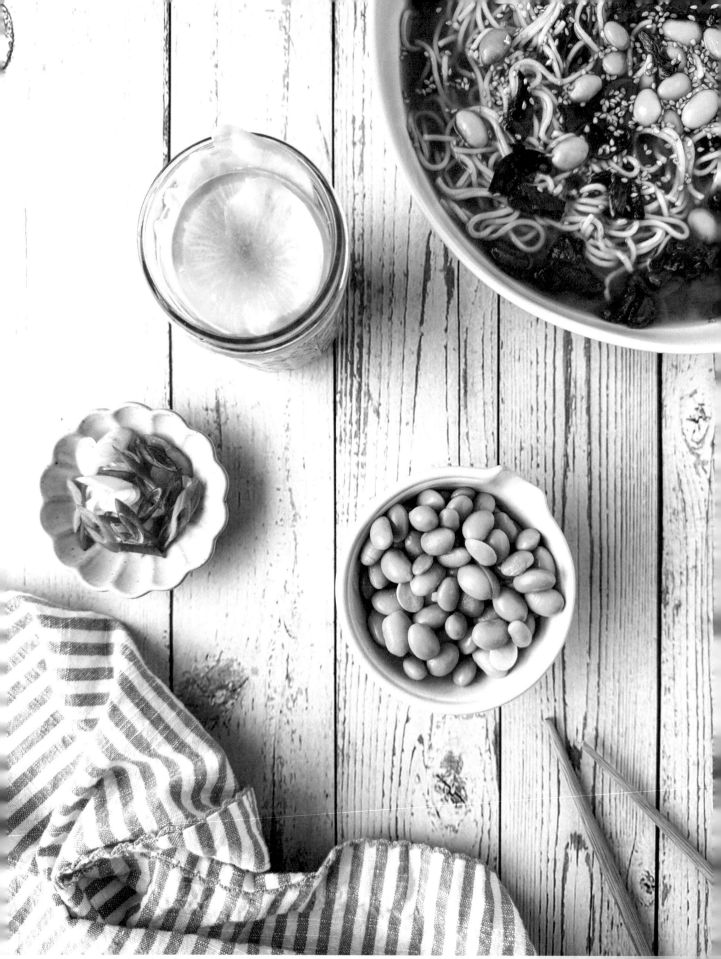

Shelled Edamame

Makes about 4 servings

Shelled edamame, also known as mukimame, are young soybeans that are quick and easy to prepare—making them one of my favorite go-to protein sources when time is tight. They're perfect tossed into salads, stir-fries, or noodle bowls, especially with Asian-inspired flavors. Look for them fresh or frozen at most grocery stores.

INGREDIENTS

- 1 (9–12-ounce) package shelled edamame, fresh or frozen

METHOD

1. Prepare according to package instructions.
2. For leftovers, allow to cool and store in an airtight container for up to 4 days.

VARIATION

Sesame Tamari Edamame: Heat the prepared edamame in a skillet over medium heat. Drizzle with 2 teaspoons of tamari and 1 teaspoon of toasted sesame oil, stirring to coat. Sauté for 2 minutes, or until warmed through.

NUTRITIONAL INFORMATION (PER SERVING)

Based on 9 ounces. Calories 77.2, Carbohydrate 3.8 g, Fiber 3.3 g, Total Sugars 1.4 g, Added Sugars 0 g, Fat 3.3 g, Saturated Fat 0.4 g, Protein 7.6 g, Sodium 3.8 mg, Iron 1.4 mg

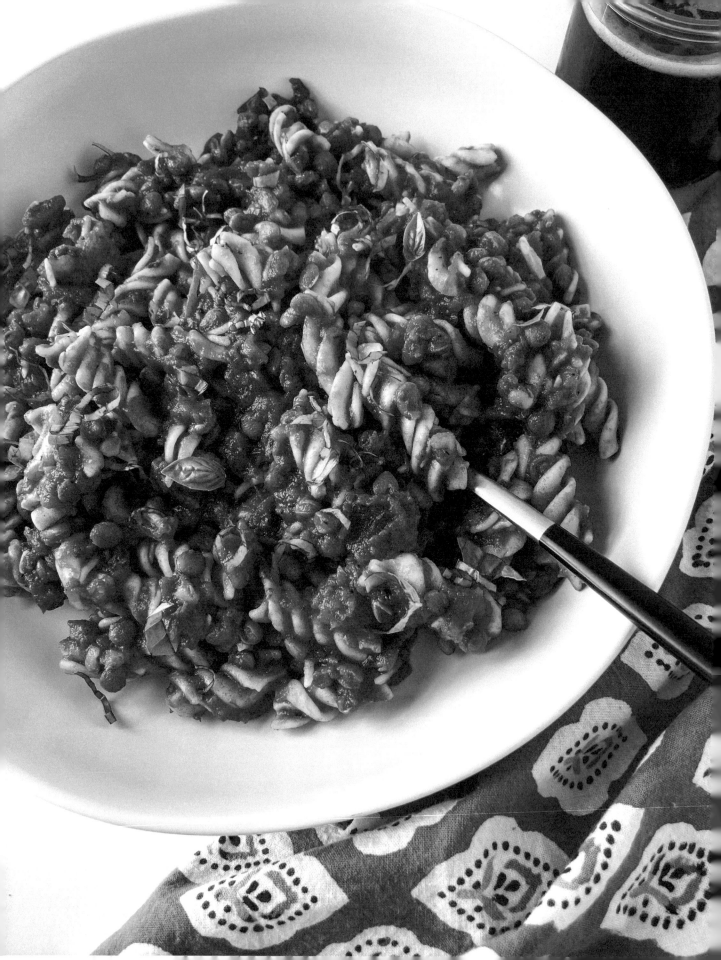

Easy Lentil Marinara

Makes about 4 servings

I love making this easy recipe on busy weeknights! Canned lentils and spices are added to marinara sauce for a quick and nutritious meal. Serve over your favorite whole-grain or legume pasta and garnish with lots of fresh basil.

INGREDIENTS

- 1 (32-ounce) jar marinara
- 1 (15-ounce) can brown or green lentils, drained and rinsed
- 1 teaspoon dried oregano
- 1 teaspoon dried thyme
- ½ cup freshly torn basil leaves

METHOD

1. In a medium saucepan, combine the marinara, lentils, oregano, and thyme, stirring until combined. Heat over medium-high heat and bring to a boil. Reduce heat to low and simmer for 10 to 12 minutes, or until warmed through.
2. Garnish with basil.

VARIATION

Add ¼ cup of your favorite hummus to the marinara mixture for added protein and creaminess.

NUTRITIONAL INFORMATION (PER SERVING)

Based on Rao's Homemade Marinara.
Calories 306.5, Carbohydrate 29.9 g, Fiber 8.5 g, Total Sugars 6.5 g, Added Sugars 0 g, Fat 16.5 g, Saturated Fat 2.1 g, Protein 11.8 g, Sodium 1016.1 mg, Iron 6.1 mg

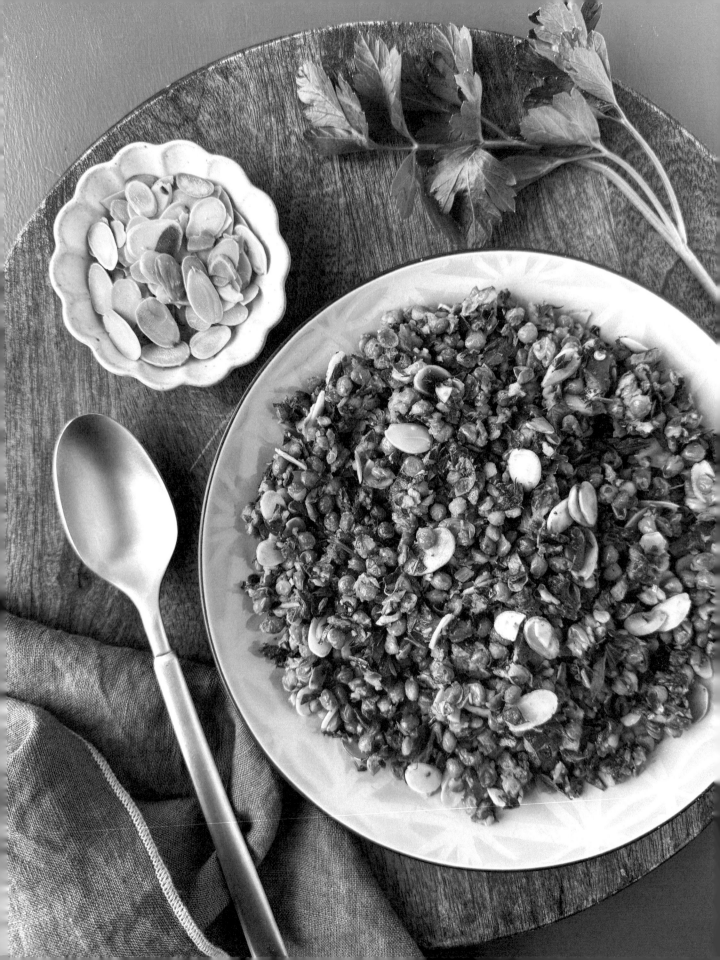

Herby Lentils with Olives

Makes about 4 servings

These Mediterranean-inspired lentils are bright, tangy, and loaded with fresh herbs. We love pairing them with Roasted Potato Cubes (page 157) or a bed of grains, or tucked into a whole-grain pita with chopped cucumbers and tomatoes.

INGREDIENTS

- 2 tablespoons extra-virgin olive oil
- ¼ cup diced red onion
- 2 medium garlic cloves, minced
- ½ teaspoon ground cumin
- ¼ teaspoon crushed red pepper flakes (optional)
- 1 (15-ounce) can green or brown lentils, rinsed and drained
- ¼ cup chopped pitted Kalamata olives
- 2 tablespoons fresh lemon juice
- ½ cup chopped fresh parsley leaves
- ½ cup chopped fresh basil leaves
- ⅓ cup toasted sliced almonds
- ⅛ teaspoon freshly ground black pepper

Tip:
This recipe is a great way to use up extra herbs that would otherwise be tossed! Cilantro, mint, or chives would also work well in this recipe.

METHOD

1. Heat the oil in a large nonstick skillet over medium heat. Add the onion and a pinch of salt and pepper and cook until soft, about 2 minutes.
2. Stir in the garlic, cumin, and red pepper flakes (if using) and cook until fragrant, about 1 minute.
3. Reduce heat to low and add the lentils, olives, and lemon juice and stir until combined. Cook for 3 minutes or until warmed through.
4. Stir in the fresh herbs and almonds. Taste and season with salt, if desired.
5. Serve immediately or at room temperature.
6. Refrigerate leftovers in an airtight container for up to 3 days.

NUTRITIONAL INFORMATION (PER SERVING)

Per serving: Calories 261.2, Carbohydrate 27.3 g, Fiber 8.3 g, Total Sugars 1.7 g, Added Sugars 0 g, Fat 12.8 g, Saturated Fat 1.6 g, Protein 12.5 g, Sodium 325.5 mg, Iron 5.8 mg

Tempeh: Different Types + How to Prepare

Tempeh is a fermented soybean product known for its firm texture and nutty flavor. It is a rich source of plant-based protein, fiber, vitamins, and minerals that is also known for its probiotic benefits, promoting gut health.

Types of Tempeh

Choose organic tempeh whenever possible, as soy is often genetically modified in the U.S. Different types of tempeh include soy-based, legume-based, mixed-grain, and flavored. For the recipes in this book, we'll be using unflavored soy-based tempeh, which is available in the refrigerated section near tofu at most markets. Its neutral flavor makes it the perfect canvas for a variety of seasonings and sauces!

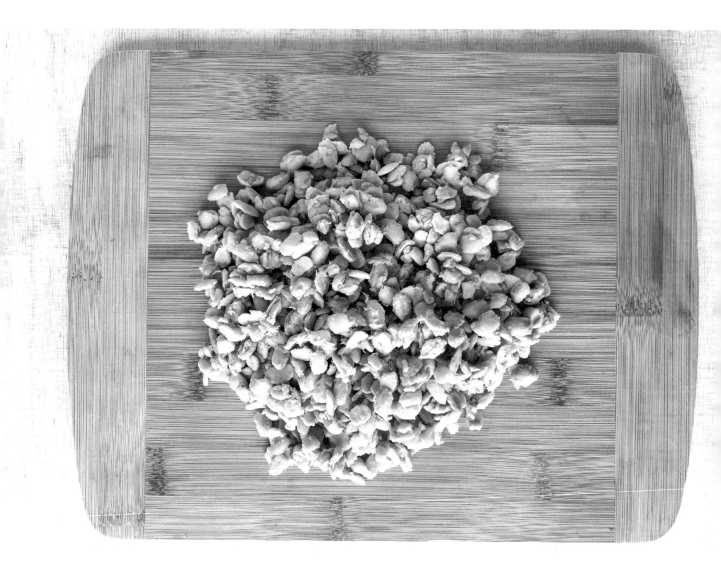

Tempeh: How to Cut

Tempeh can be cut into many different shapes, like strips, triangles, and cubes. Our go-to method is cubed tempeh, which can be added to bowls, wraps, and salads.

1. Remove the packaging and place the tempeh block on a cutting board.
2. Slice lengthwise into ½-inch strips.
3. Rotate the strips 90 degrees, then cut them into evenly sized cubes.

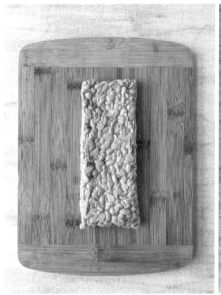 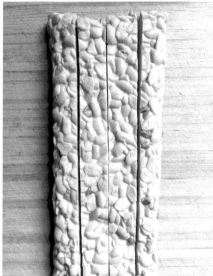 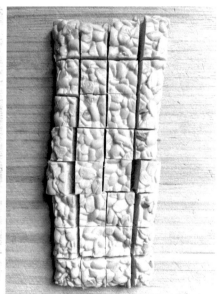

Tempeh: How to Crumble

Use your hands to crumble into individual soybeans.

Tempeh: How to Marinate

Place your marinade ingredients in a medium bowl or storage container and whisk until combined. Add the tempeh to the marinade and toss until evenly coated. Cover and refrigerate for a minimum of 15 minutes, or overnight for best results.

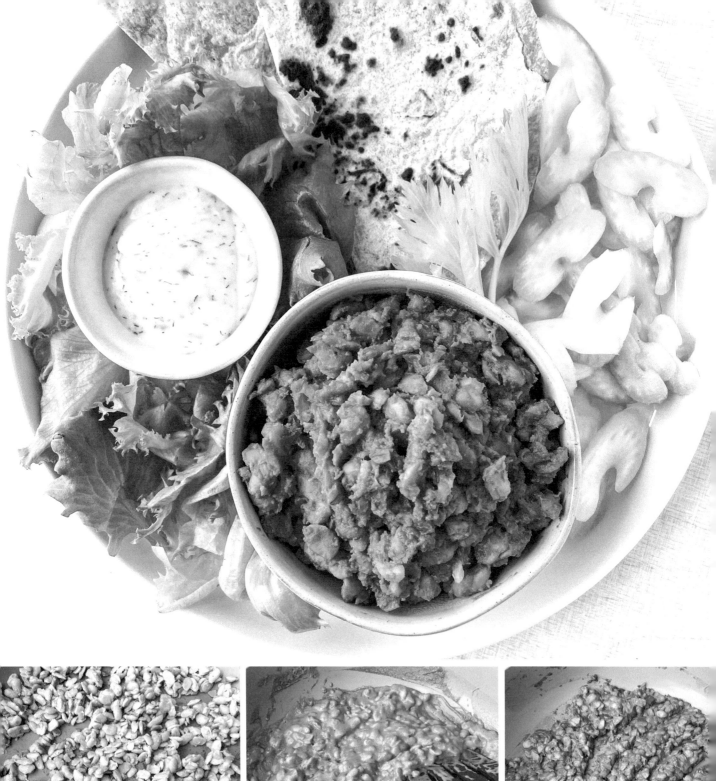

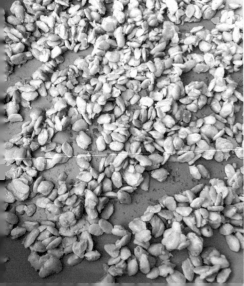
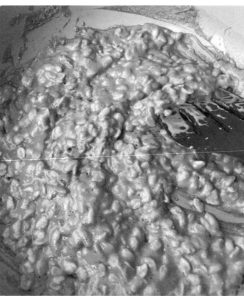
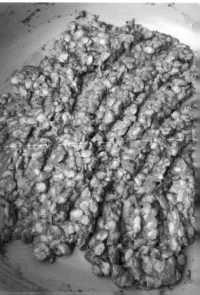

Buffalo Tempeh Crumbles

Makes about 4 servings

....

Crumbled tempeh is sautéed and cooked in a butter-free buffalo sauce, creating a flavorful and protein-packed dish. Serve Buffalo Tempeh Crumbles in a whole-grain wrap or on a bed of whole grains, topped with crunchy celery and drizzled with Dill Sauce (page 55).

INGREDIENTS

- 2 (8-ounce) blocks of tempeh, crumbled
- 1 teaspoon extra-virgin olive oil

BUFFALO SAUCE

- ⅓ cup Frank's RedHot Original Cayenne Pepper Sauce
- ⅓ cup water
- 3 tablespoons raw cashews
- 2 tablespoons reduced-sodium tamari
- ¾ tablespoon pure maple syrup
- 2 teaspoons white wine vinegar
- 1 teaspoon garlic powder

Tip:
Instead of tempeh, use a block of extra-firm or super-firm tofu that has been crumbled.

METHOD

1. Make the sauce: Combine all the ingredients in a high-speed blender and blend until smooth and creamy. If using a regular blender, soak the cashews in hot water for 15 minutes and discard the soaking water. Proceed with the recipe as directed.

2. Prep the tempeh: Rinse and dry the tempeh. Gently crumble into small pieces using your hands.

3. Sauté: Heat oil in a large nonstick skillet over medium-high heat. Once shimmering, add the crumbled tempeh and sauté until lightly golden, stirring frequently, about 2 minutes.

4. Reduce heat to medium-low and add the buffalo sauce and stir until the tempeh is coated. Simmer for 6 to 8 minutes or until the sauce has reduced and clings to the tempeh, stirring occasionally.

5. Refrigerate cooled leftovers in an airtight container for up to 7 days.

NUTRITIONAL INFORMATION (PER SERVING)

Per serving: Calories 279, Carbohydrate 14.1 g, Fiber 4.5 g, Total Sugars 5.9 g, Added Sugars 2.2 g, Fat 16.1 g, Saturated Fat 3.5 g, Protein 25.2 g, Sodium 1122.9 mg, Iron 3.7 mg

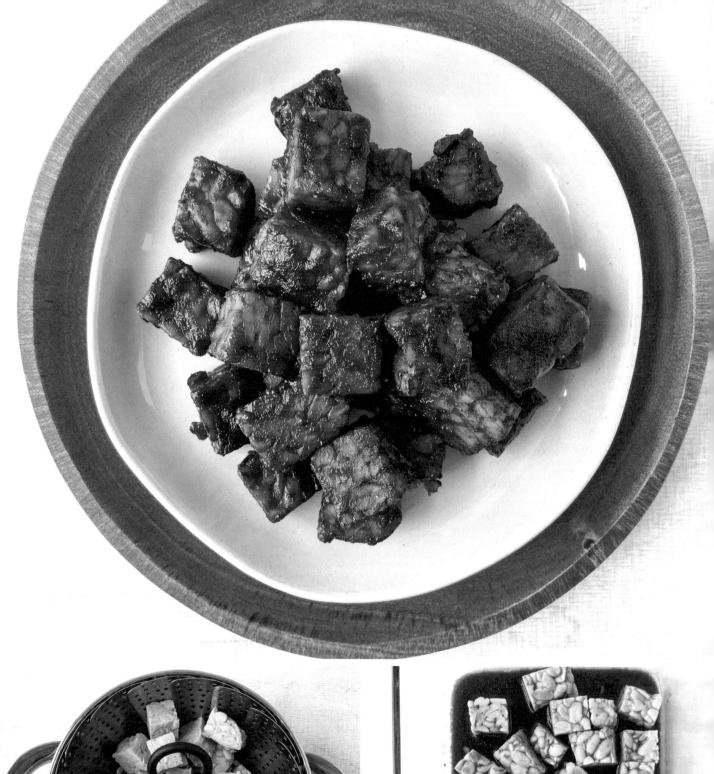
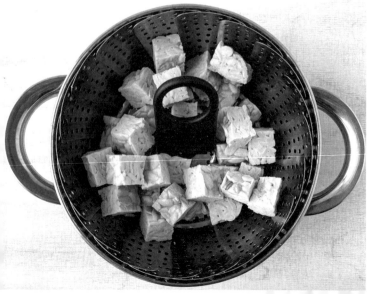
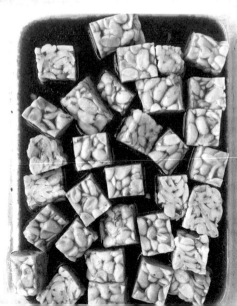

Asian Tempeh Cubes

Makes about 4 servings

Tempeh cubes are steamed, marinated, and sautéed with a tasty umami sauce. Combine these saucy tempeh cubes with rice noodles and your favorite stir-fried veggies.

INGREDIENTS

- 1 (8-ounce) block of tempeh, cubed
- 3 tablespoons reduced-sodium tamari
- 1 tablespoon rice vinegar
- 1 tablespoon pure maple syrup
- 1 teaspoon sriracha
- 1 teaspoon sesame oil
- 1 teaspoon arrowroot starch (or cornstarch)

NUTRITIONAL INFORMATION (PER SERVING)

Per serving: Calories 144.4, Carbohydrate 9.3 g, Fiber 2.2 g, Total Sugars 5 g, Added Sugars 3.2 g, Fat 7.3 g, Saturated Fat 1.6 g, Protein 13 g, Sodium 565.7 mg, Iron 1.9 mg

METHOD

1. Prepare the tempeh: Cut the tempeh into approximately ¾-inch cubes. Add a steamer basket to a medium saucepan with 1 inch of water. Bring the water to a simmer and add the tempeh. Cover and steam for 10 minutes. This will soften the tempeh so it will absorb more flavor from the marinade.

2. Make the marinade: In the meantime, in a shallow dish, combine the tamari, vinegar, maple syrup, sriracha, sesame oil, and arrowroot/cornstarch and whisk until combined without clumps. Carefully add the steamed tempeh and toss until evenly coated. Marinate for a minimum of 20 minutes.

3. Sauté: Heat a medium nonstick skillet over medium-low heat. Using a slotted spoon, remove the tempeh cubes from the marinade and add to the warm skillet in a single layer. Cook for 2 to 3 minutes until some sides are golden brown, stirring frequently.

4. Pour the remaining marinade into the skillet and toss until the tempeh is evenly coated. Cook until the sauce thickens, about 2 minutes.

5. For leftovers, allow to cool and refrigerate in an airtight container for up to 7 days.

BASES

Whole Grains
+
Starches

Carbohydrates are your body's preferred fuel source, and it's okay to eat them! However, not all carbohydrates are created equal.

Refined grains are the number one source of calories in the average American diet. When choosing carbohydrates, opt for the least refined versions to stay full longer, support blood sugar control, and promote a healthy weight.

- Cilantro Lime Rice
- Turmeric Rice
- Mediterranean Quinoa
- Farro
- Sweet Potato Boats
- Roasted Potato Cubes
- Noodles: Whole Grains + Legumes
- Handhelds: Wraps, Pita + Bread

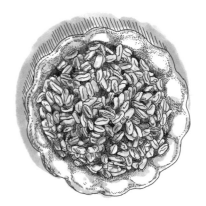

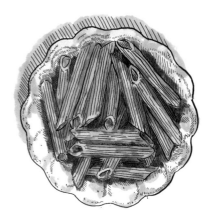

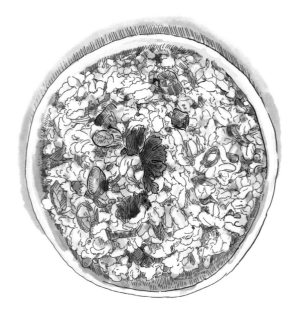

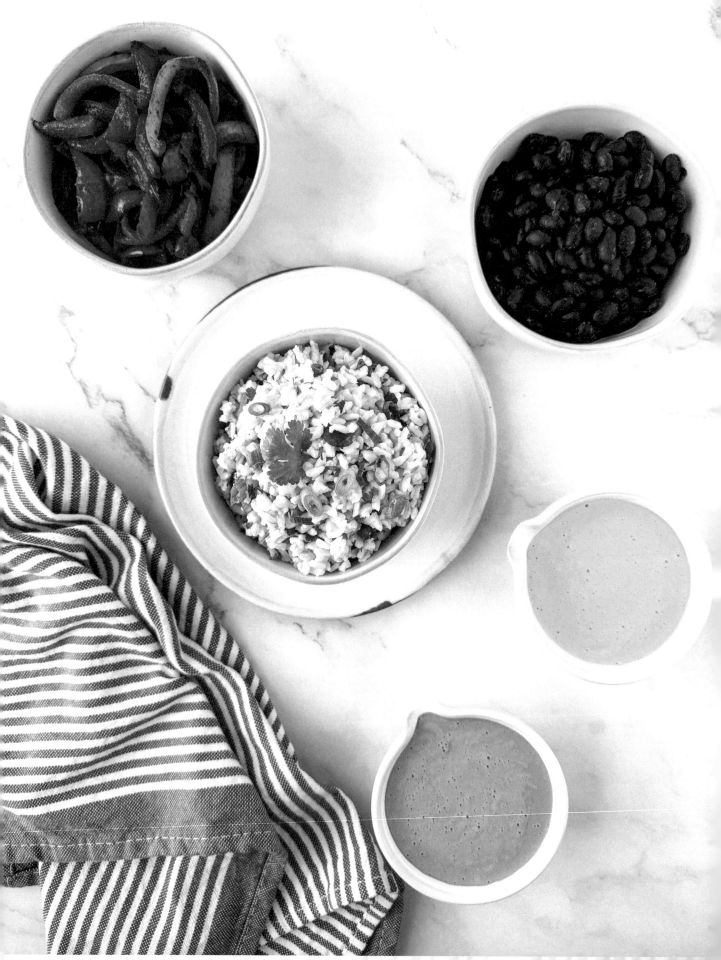

Cilantro Lime Rice

Makes about 6 servings

Brown rice mixed with green onion, cilantro, and fresh lime juice creates a bright and hearty base or side dish. It's a perfect match for Asian- and Latin-inspired nourish bowls.

INGREDIENTS

- 1 cup dry basmati brown rice, rinsed and drained
- 1 green onion, thinly sliced
- 2 tablespoons fresh lime juice
- 1 medium garlic clove, minced
- ½ teaspoon lime zest
- 2 teaspoons extra-virgin olive oil (optional)
- ½ cup finely chopped cilantro leaves
- ¼ teaspoon salt, or to taste

METHOD

1. Cook the rice according to package instructions.
2. Uncover and fluff the rice with a fork. Stir in the green onion, lime juice, garlic, lime zest, oil (if using), and salt. Let cool for 5 minutes.
3. Gently stir in the cilantro.
4. For leftovers, allow to cool and refrigerate in an airtight container for up to 5 days.

NUTRITIONAL INFORMATION (PER SERVING)

Per serving: Calories 129.2, Carbohydrate 24.2 g, Fiber 1.2 g, Total Sugars 0.4 g, Added Sugars 0 g, Fat 2.5 g, Saturated Fat 0.4 g, Protein 2.4 g, Sodium 100.9 mg, Iron 0.5 mg

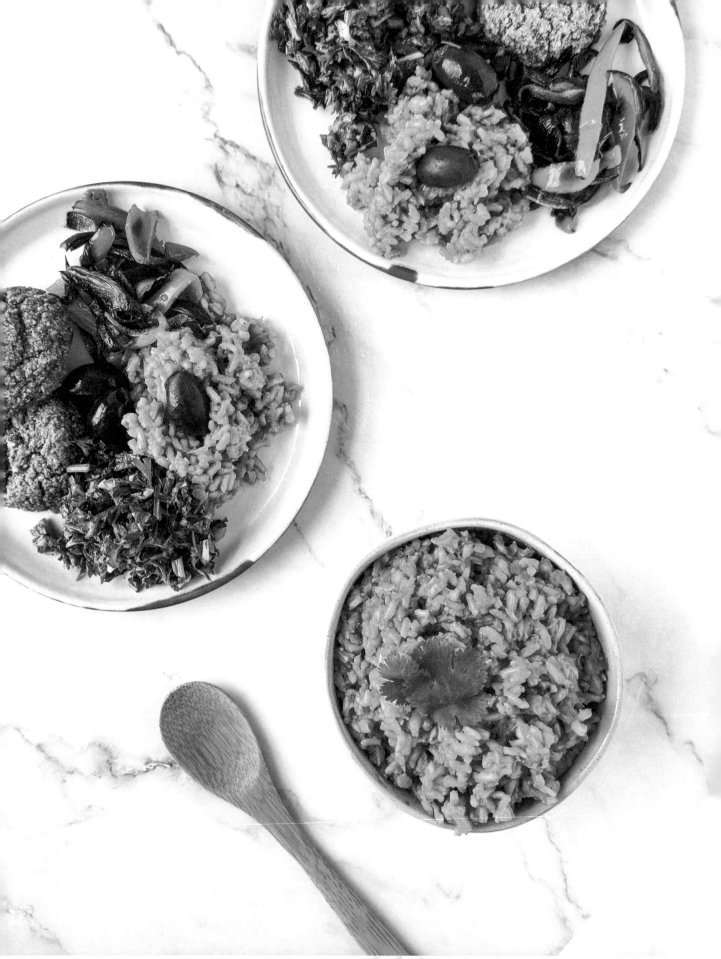

Turmeric Rice

Makes about 6 servings

This golden, earthy rice is infused with ginger, garlic, and turmeric creating a nutritious and savory base or side dish. Perfect for pairing with Mediterranean-, Cajun-, and Indian-inspired dishes.

INGREDIENTS

- 1 teaspoon extra-virgin olive oil
- ¼ cup finely diced yellow onion
- 2 teaspoons minced fresh ginger
- ½ teaspoon turmeric powder
- 2 medium garlic cloves, minced
- ⅛ teaspoon freshly ground black pepper
- 1 cup dry brown basmati rice, rinsed and drained
- 2 cups low-sodium vegetable broth
- 1 bay leaf

METHOD

1. In a medium saucepan, heat oil over medium heat. Once shimmering, add the onion and sauté until translucent, about 3 minutes.
2. Add the ginger, turmeric, garlic, and pepper and cook until fragrant, about 1 minute.
3. Reduce heat to medium-low and stir in the rice until coated with spices. Stirring frequently, cook until the edges start to turn golden, about 5 minutes.
4. Add the broth and bay leaf, and bring to a boil. Cover and reduce heat to low and simmer for 35 to 45 minutes, or until the liquid has been absorbed and the rice is tender (refer to the rice package instructions for timing).
5. Remove from heat and keep covered for 10 minutes. Fluff with a fork and season with salt and pepper, if desired.
6. For leftovers, allow to cool and refrigerate in an airtight container for up to 4 days, or freeze for up to 2 months.

NUTRITIONAL INFORMATION (PER SERVING)

Per serving: Calories 119.5, Carbohydrate 24.7 g, Fiber 1.8 g, Total Sugars 1.5 g, Added Sugars 0.4 g, Fat 1.9 g, Saturated Fat 0.2 g, Protein 3.1 g, Sodium 46 mg, Iron 1.1 mg

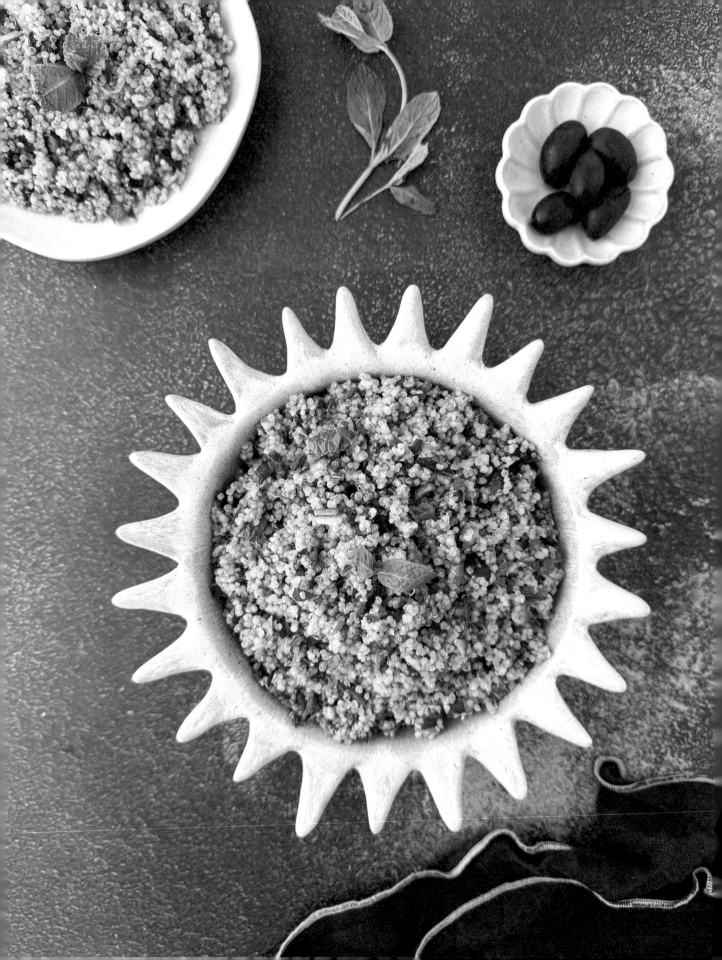

Mediterranean Quinoa

Makes about 6 servings

Chilled quinoa is tossed with fresh herbs, olives, onions, and a splash of lemon juice, making it a versatile option as a main dish, side, or nourish bowl base.

INGREDIENTS

- 1 cup dry quinoa
- 2 tablespoons fresh lemon juice
- 1 tablespoon extra-virgin olive oil
- ¼ teaspoon salt, or to taste
- ⅛ teaspoon freshly ground black pepper
- ½ cup sliced pitted Kalamata olives
- ¼ cup finely diced red onion
- ½ cup chopped fresh mint leaves
- ½ cup chopped fresh parsley leaves

METHOD

1. Cook the quinoa according to package directions. Allow to cool.
2. In a large bowl, combine the lemon juice, oil, salt, pepper, olives, and onion until evenly coated.
3. Stir in the cooled quinoa and herbs until well combined.
4. For leftovers, refrigerate in an airtight container for up to 3 days.

NUTRITIONAL INFORMATION (PER SERVING)

Per serving: Calories 146.8, Carbohydrate 21 g, Fiber 3 g, Total Sugars 2.4 g, Added Sugars 0 g, Fat 5.3 g, Saturated Fat 0.8 g, Protein 4.6 g, Sodium 187.9 mg, Iron 3.3 mg

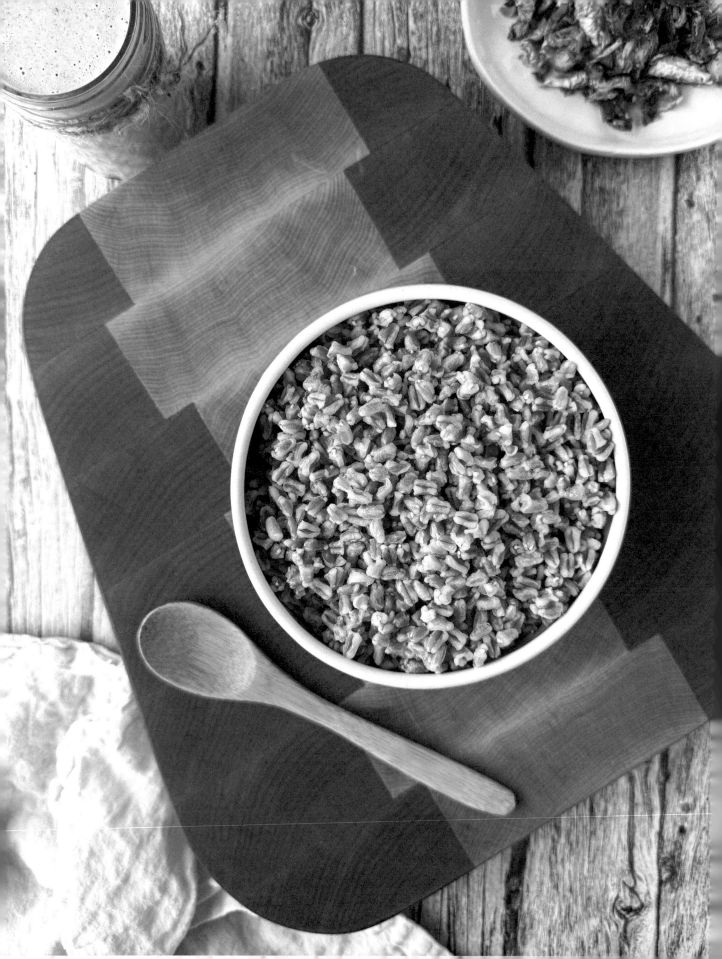

Farro

With its nutty flavor and chewy texture, this ancient whole grain is perfect for salads. Farro also shines in soups, nourish bowls, or as a wholesome side dish.

INGREDIENTS

- 1 cup dry farro
- Water

METHOD

1. Cook according to the package directions.
2. For leftovers, allow to cool and refrigerate in an airtight container for up to 5 days or freeze for up to 2 months.

NUTRITIONAL INFORMATION (PER SERVING)

Per serving: Calories 113.4, Carbohydrate 24.7 g, Fiber 4.2 g, Total Sugars 0.1 g, Added Sugars 0 g, Fat 0.5 g, Saturated Fat 0.1 g, Protein 4.4 g, Sodium 0.7 mg, Iron 1.1 mg

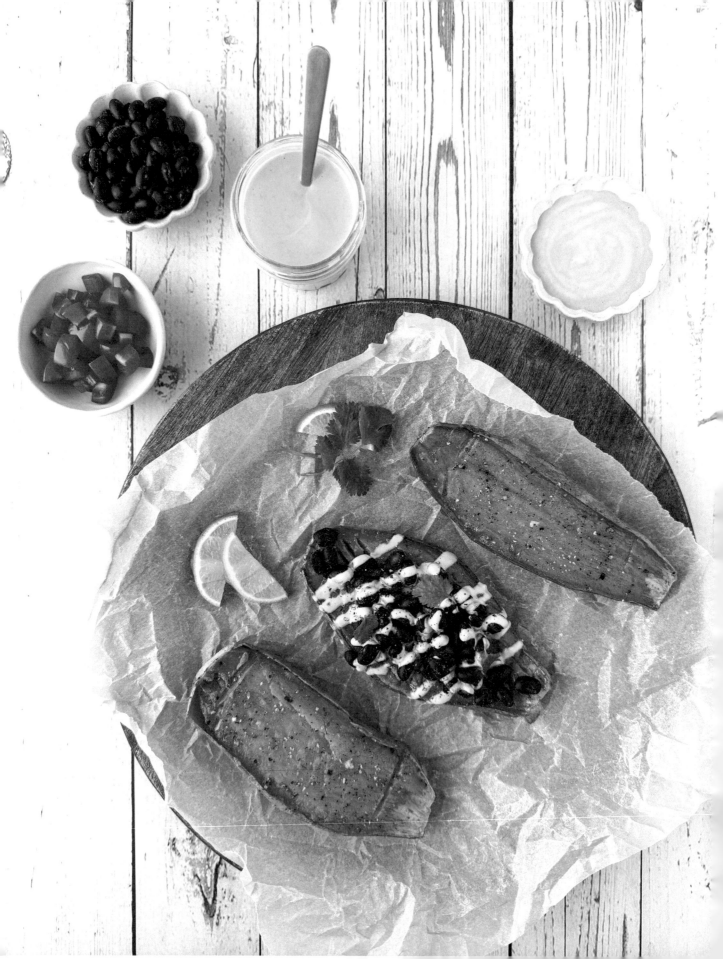

Sweet Potato Boats

Makes about 8 servings

Soft and caramelized, sweet potato boats make a delicious and hearty base for stuffed creations! Pair them with roasted cauliflower and Buffalo Sauce (page 35) or top with Easy Black Beans (page 111) and Cashew Queso (page 75).

INGREDIENTS

- 4 medium sweet potatoes, cut in half, lengthwise
- 1 tablespoon extra-virgin olive oil
- ⅛ teaspoon salt
- ⅛ teaspoon freshly ground black pepper

Tip:
Instead of sweet potatoes, use Japanese sweet potatoes, russet potatoes, or Yukon Gold potatoes. Cooking times will vary based on size.

METHOD

1. Preheat oven to 425°F. Line a large rimmed baking sheet with parchment paper.
2. Place the potatoes on the baking sheet and drizzle with oil and sprinkle with salt and pepper. Massage each potato until evenly coated and place cut-side down.
3. Cook on the middle oven rack for 35 to 45 minutes, or until fork-tender and the flesh side starts to brown. Rotate the baking sheet 180 degrees after the first 20 minutes.
4. Allow to cool for 5 minutes. If you are stuffing the potatoes, mash the flesh with the back of a fork while still warm. Add your favorite toppings and sauce, if desired.
5. Refrigerate leftovers in an airtight container for up to a week.

NUTRITIONAL INFORMATION (PER SERVING)

Per serving: Calories 70.9, Carbohydrate 13.1 g, Fiber 2 g, Total Sugars 2.7 g, Added Sugars 0 g, Fat 1.7 g, Saturated Fat 0.2 g, Protein 1 g, Sodium 72.6 mg, Iron 0.4 mg

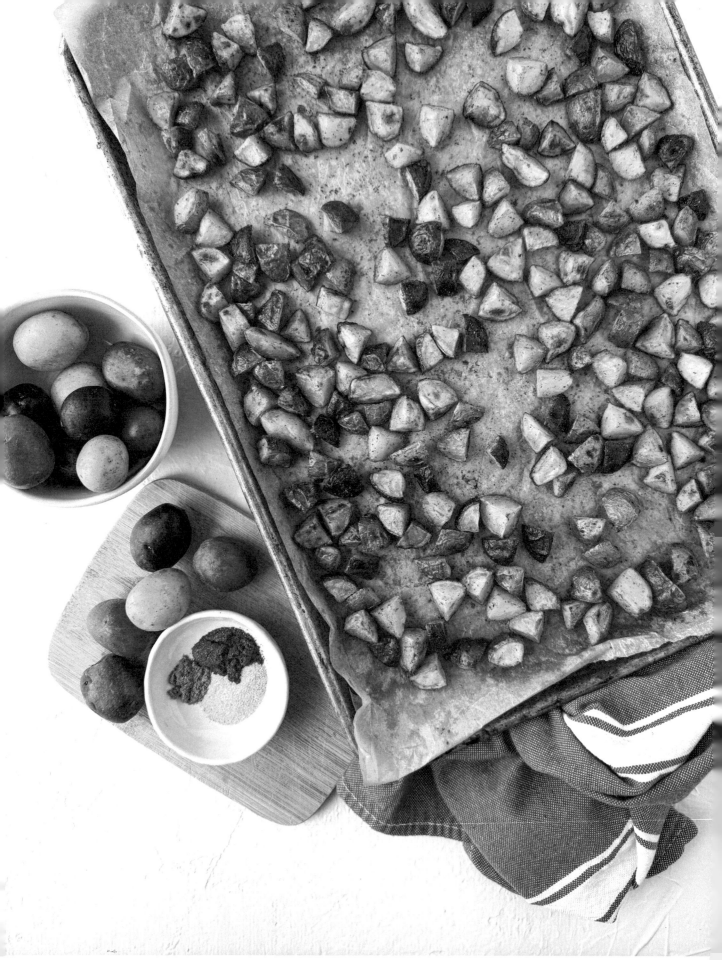

Roasted Potato Cubes

Makes about 8 servings

These seasoned, roasted potato cubes are perfect for meal prep! Savor them warm in nourish bowls and tacos, or toss them into hearty salads with a drizzle of Sweet Dijon Dressing (page 33) or Creamy Cilantro Dressing (page 73).

INGREDIENTS

- 2 pounds sweet or baby potatoes, cut into ½-inch cubes
- 1 tablespoon extra-virgin olive oil
- 1 teaspoon garlic powder
- 1 teaspoon paprika
- ¼ teaspoon ground cumin
- ¼ teaspoon salt

Tips:
Boost nutrients and plant diversity by experimenting with colorful potatoes! Try a mix of blue, red, and yellow baby potatoes, or combine purple and orange sweet potatoes.

Leave the peel on whenever possible to increase the fiber and protein content.

METHOD

1. Place the cubed potatoes in a bowl of cold water and soak for 30 minutes. Drain and pat dry with a dish towel to remove excess moisture.
2. Preheat oven to 425°F. Line two rimmed baking sheets with parchment paper.
3. In a large bowl, toss the potato cubes with oil and dried spices until evenly coated.
4. Spread half the potatoes on each baking sheet in a single layer. Avoid overcrowding to ensure crispiness instead of steaming.
5. Place on the middle rack and cook for 30 to 35 minutes, flipping after 20 minutes, until tender and golden brown at the edges.
6. Season with additional salt if desired.
7. Refrigerate cooled leftovers in an airtight container for up to 5 days.

NUTRITIONAL INFORMATION (PER SERVING)

Per serving: Calories 114, Carbohydrate 23.1 g, Fiber 3.5 g, Total Sugars 4.7 g, Added Sugars 0 g, Fat 1.8 g, Saturated Fat 0.3 g, Protein 1.9 g, Sodium 136.1 mg, Iron 0.8 mg

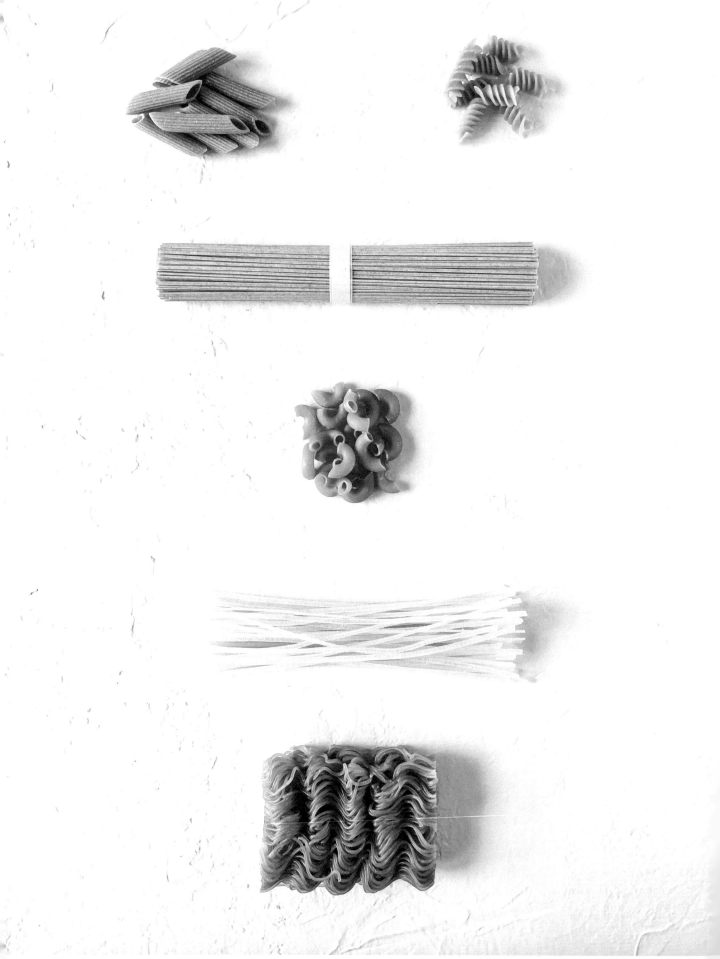

NOODLES: WHOLE GRAINS + LEGUMES

Noodles make a quick, versatile base for plant-based meals. With new options emerging constantly, explore and experiment to find your favorites. Here's a quick guide to our top picks:

- **Whole wheat pasta:** Made with durum whole wheat flour.
- **Brown rice and quinoa pasta:** A gluten-free favorite that holds its shape well. Made with brown rice, quinoa flour, and water.
- **Buckwheat soba noodles:** Made with buckwheat flour. Nutty and hearty, great for soups or stir-fries.
- **Legume pasta:** Chickpea and lentil varieties pack protein and fiber. Made with red lentil or chickpea flour.
- **Millet and brown rice ramen:** A wholesome spin on classic ramen. Made with brown rice flour and millet flour.

HANDHELDS: WRAPS, PITA + BREAD

Tortillas, wraps, bread, and pita provide a quick, easy base for your favorite ingredients for grab-and-go meals. Check ingredient labels to avoid artificial additives and enriched flours. Here are some of our favorite wholesome options:

- **Tortillas and wraps:** Made with flours like 100% whole wheat, masa harina, almond, cassava root, or nutrient-rich ancient grains such as kamut and spelt.
- **Sourdough bread:** Made with flour, water, salt, and a sourdough starter.
- **Sprouted bread:** Packed with nutrients from sprouted whole grains and legumes.
- **Whole wheat pita:** A simple mix of whole wheat flour, water, yeast, and salt.

Tip:
When available, choose non-GMO options for whole wheat, corn, and chickpea products as these are often GMO products in the U.S.

NUTS

+

SEEDS

Nuts and seeds are tiny powerhouses, packed with healthy fats, vitamins, and minerals. While nuts are more calorically dense than many other plant foods, studies show they do not contribute to weight gain.[2][3][4]

Just ¼ cup of nuts per day may help reduce the risk of death from heart disease, stroke, cancer, respiratory disease, and diabetes.[5]

- Almond Parmesan
- Chili Roasted Mixed Nuts
- Seedy Nut Butter

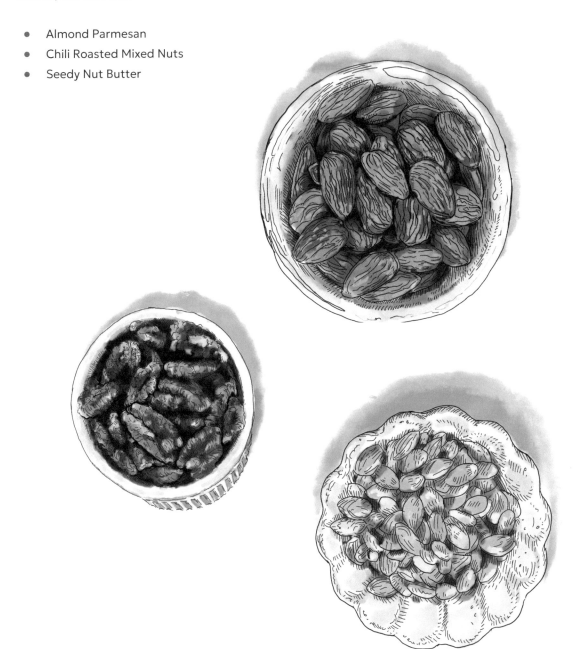

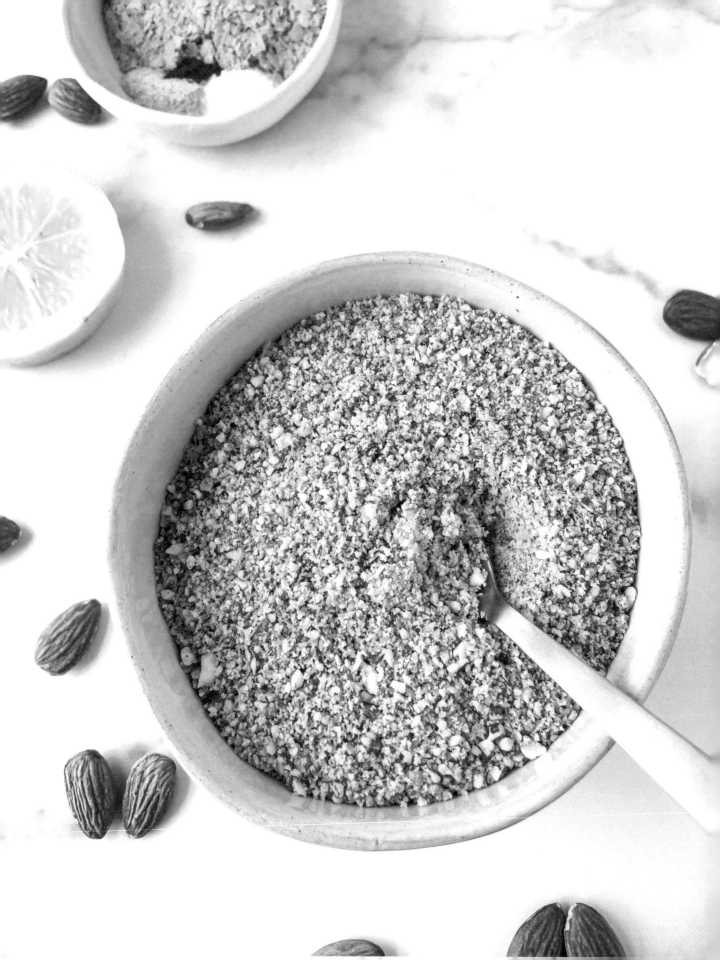

Almond Parmesan

Makes about 4 servings

Enhance your dishes with a deliciously cheesy, nutty flavor using this dairy-free Parmesan! Sprinkle on pasta, soups, salads, and more for a touch of umami goodness.

INGREDIENTS

- ½ cup raw almonds, unsalted
- 2 ½ tablespoons nutritional yeast
- 1 teaspoon fresh lemon juice
- ½ teaspoon salt
- ¼ teaspoon garlic powder
- Pinch smoked paprika

METHOD

1. Combine all the ingredients in a food processor with the S-blade. Process into a crumbly powder, about 2 minutes. Scrape sides as needed.
2. Refrigerate in an airtight container for up to 2 months.

NUTRITIONAL INFORMATION (PER SERVING)

Per serving: Calories 107.5, Carbohydrate 5 g, Fiber 2.7 g, Total Sugars 0.7 g, Added Sugars 0 g, Fat 8.1 g, Saturated Fat 0.6 g, Protein 5.4 g, Sodium 301.3 mg, Iron 0.8 mg

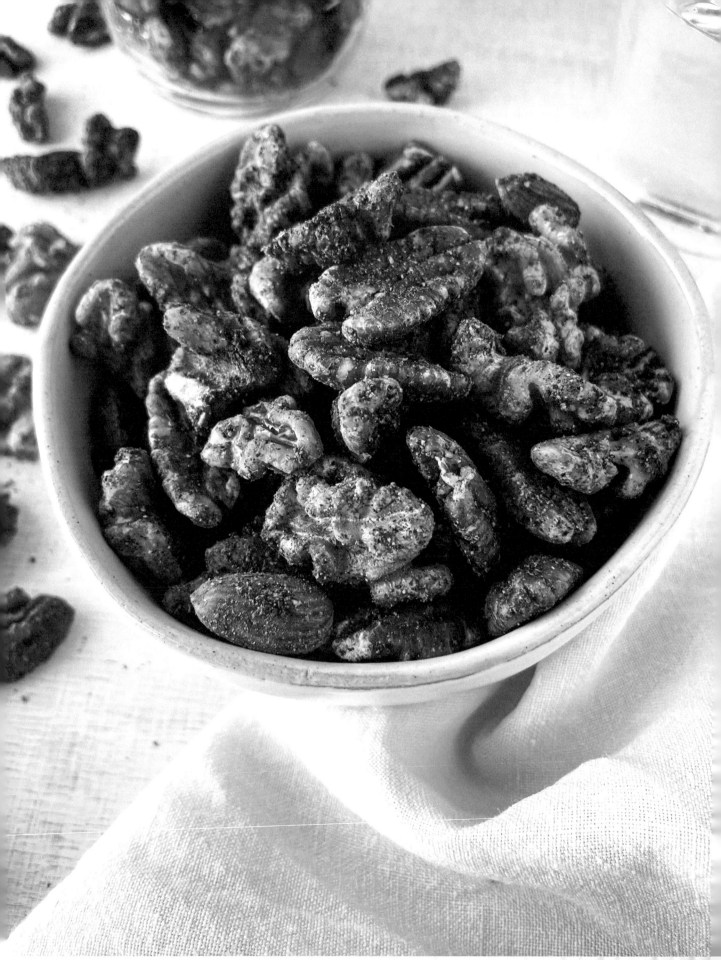

Chili Roasted Mixed Nuts

Makes about 16 servings

Savory with a touch of sweetness, these chili-roasted nuts make a perfect grab-and-go snack or a flavorful addition to a grazing board for game day or the holidays.

INGREDIENTS

- 2 cups raw walnuts
- 1 cup raw pecans
- 1 cup raw almonds
- 1 tablespoon extra-virgin olive oil
- 1 tablespoon pure maple syrup
- 1 tablespoon plus 1 teaspoon chili powder
- 1 teaspoon garlic powder
- ½ teaspoon ground cumin
- ½ teaspoon salt
- ¼ teaspoon cayenne (more if you like it spicy)

METHOD

1. Preheat oven to 350°F. Line a rimmed baking sheet with parchment paper.
2. In a large bowl, combine the nuts, oil, and maple syrup. Stir until evenly coated.
3. In a small bowl, mix together all the spices. Sprinkle over the nut mixture and stir until evenly coated.
4. Spread nut mixture on the prepared baking sheet in an even layer.
5. Bake on the middle rack for 13 to 15 minutes, or until lightly golden, flipping once after 8 minutes. Since oven temperatures can vary, keep an eye on the nuts around the 13-minute mark to prevent burning.
6. Allow to cool completely. Store in an airtight container for up to 2 weeks, or freeze for up to 2 months.

NUTRITIONAL INFORMATION (PER SERVING)

Per serving: Calories 189.4, Carbohydrate 5.8 g, Fiber 2.8 g, Total Sugars 1.8 g, Added Sugars 0.7 g, Fat 18.1 g, Saturated Fat 1.6 g, Protein 4.4 g, Sodium 93.5 mg, Iron 1 mg

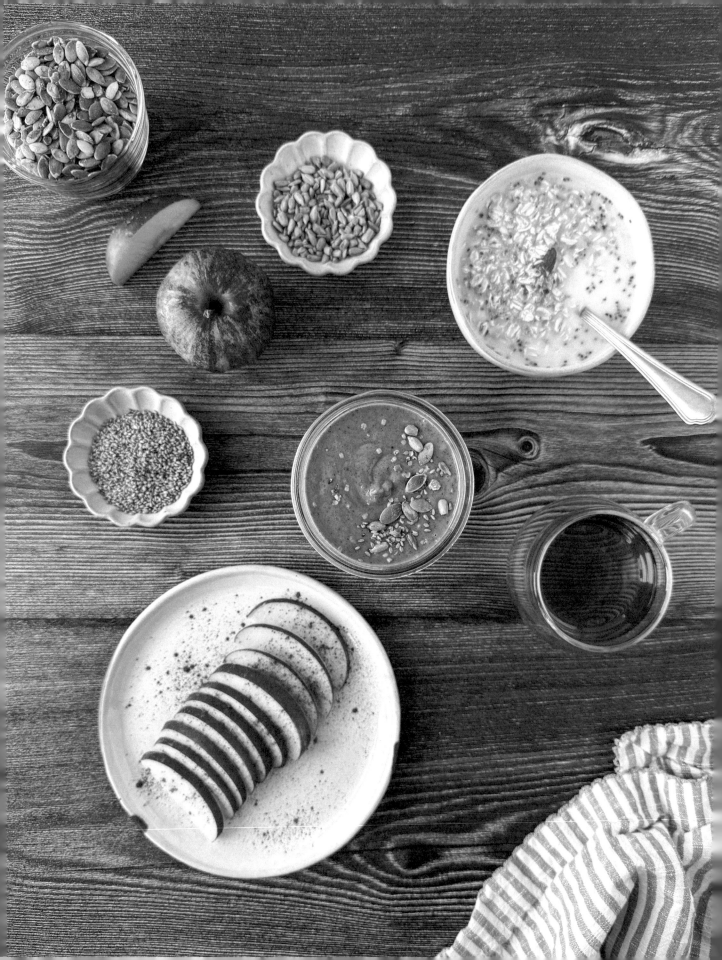

Seedy Nut Butter

Makes about 30 servings

This savory, crunchy spread makes the perfect topper for overnight oats and oatmeal, or enjoy it as a dip with cinnamon-dusted apples or banana slices for a quick snack or wholesome dessert. Packed with protein, fiber, omega fatty acids, and healthy fats, it's a simple way to elevate both flavor and nutrition.

INGREDIENTS

- 1 ½ cups smooth peanut butter, almond butter, or cashew butter
- ¼ cup roasted pepitas or sunflower seeds
- 3 tablespoons flaxseed meal, toasted sesame seeds, hemp hearts, or chia seeds

METHOD

1. In a medium bowl, mix the nut butter with your seeds of choice until evenly combined.
2. Transfer to an airtight container and store in the refrigerator for up to a month.
3. Add 1 or 2 tablespoons to your desired breakfast or fruit.

Tip:
Opt for a runny-
textured nut butter
at room temperature
for easier mixing when
combining with
the seeds.

BREAKFAST

Two of our favorite breakfasts include smoothies and savory tofu scrambles. Both include a base recipe with several variations that can be customized to your individual taste preferences. Both meals are meal-prep friendly, making mornings hassle-free!

How to Build a Smoothie

- Blueberry Cherry Smoothie
- Tropical Smoothie
- Funky Monkey Smoothie

Tofu Scramble: 3 Ways

- Southwest Scramble
- Mediterranean Scramble
- Leftover Veggie Scramble

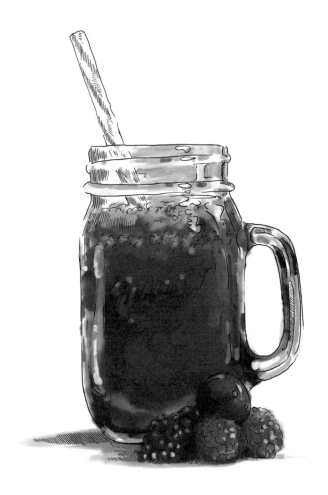

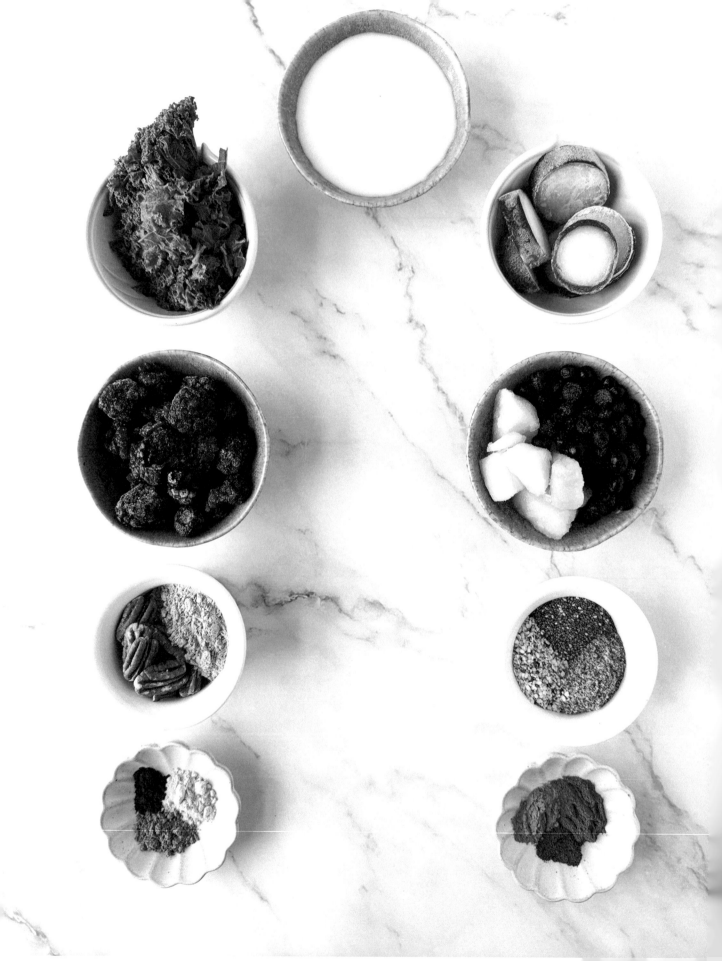

How to Build a Smoothie

Smoothies are a simple, delicious way to boost your intake of fruits, vegetables, nuts, and seeds. Use these guidelines to create a smoothie with ingredients you love! You'll also find three of our favorite smoothie recipes to get you started.

Makes 1 serving

LIQUID
1 cup

- Unsweetened nondairy milk (soy, almond, oat, cashew, coconut milk)
- Water as needed

VEGGIES
up to 2 cups,
fresh or frozen

- Organic baby spinach, organic kale, power greens
- Cauliflower, zucchini, carrots, beets (2-4 tbsp)

FRUIT
up to 1 cup,
fresh or frozen

- Wild blueberries, organic strawberries, mixed berries, cherries, apples, oranges (1 cup)
- Pineapple, mango, banana (½ cup)

**HEALTHY FATS
+ PROTEIN**
1–2 tbsp

- Plant-based protein powder
- Nut or seed butter
- Raw seeds (flaxseed meal, hemp hearts, chia seeds, sunflower seeds, pepitas)
- Raw nuts (walnuts, pecans, almonds, cashews)
- Avocado

**ADD-INS
(OPTIONAL)**
¼–1 tsp

- Spirulina, maca powder, mushroom powder, acai powder (½-1 tsp)
- Ground turmeric, ground cinnamon, a pinch of ground cloves (¼ tsp)

Smoothie Recipes Makes 1 serving

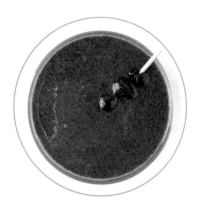

Blueberry Cherry Smoothie

- 1 cup unsweetened oat milk
- 1 cup organic kale
- ⅔ cup frozen wild blueberries
- ⅓ cup frozen cherries
- 1 tablespoon flaxseed meal
- 1 serving plant-based protein powder (vanilla or chocolate)
- Water and ice as needed

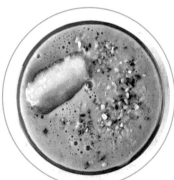

Tropical Smoothie

- 1 cup unsweetened soy milk
- 1 cup organic baby spinach
- 1 cup frozen pineapple chunks
- ½ frozen banana
- 1 tablespoon hemp hearts
- 1 serving vanilla plant-based protein powder
- Water and ice as needed

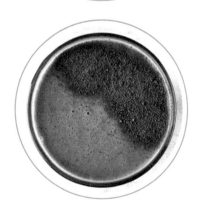

Funky Monkey Smoothie

- 1 cup unsweetened almond milk
- ½ cup frozen cauliflower
- 1 small frozen banana
- 2 tablespoons peanut butter (or almond butter)
- 1 serving chocolate plant-based protein powder
- 1 teaspoon vanilla extract
- ½ teaspoon ground cinnamon

METHOD

1. In a high-speed blender, combine the liquid with the remaining ingredients. Add water to just cover the ingredients to aid in blending. If you prefer extra-cold smoothies, add 3 to 5 ice cubes.

2. Blend until smooth and creamy. Taste and adjust. If more sweetness is desired, add a ½ ripe banana, two dates, or 1 teaspoon of raw honey. Enjoy!

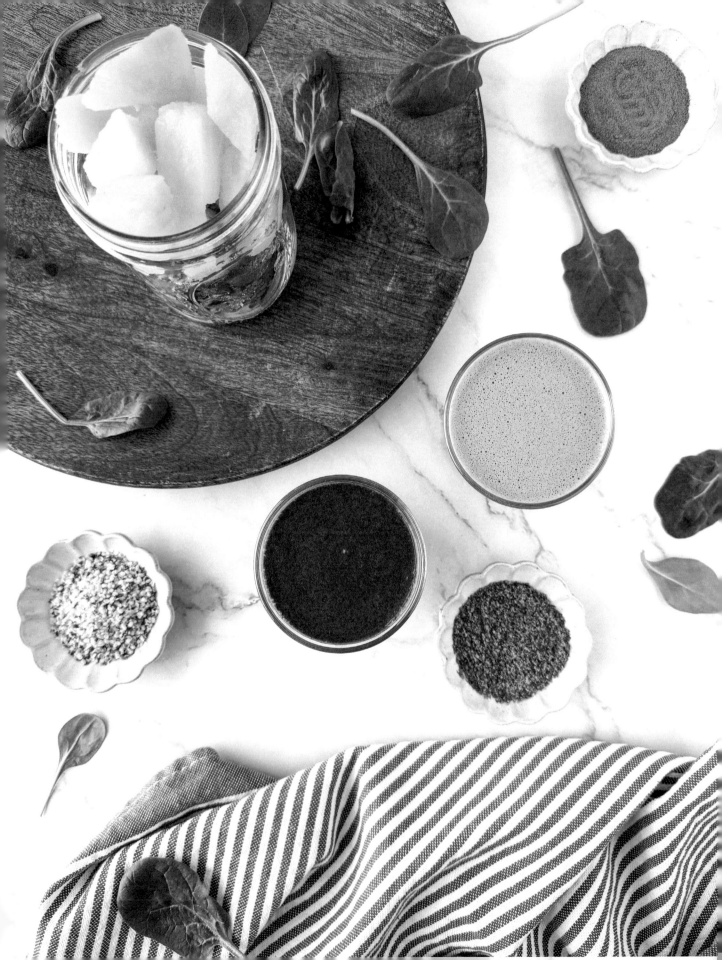

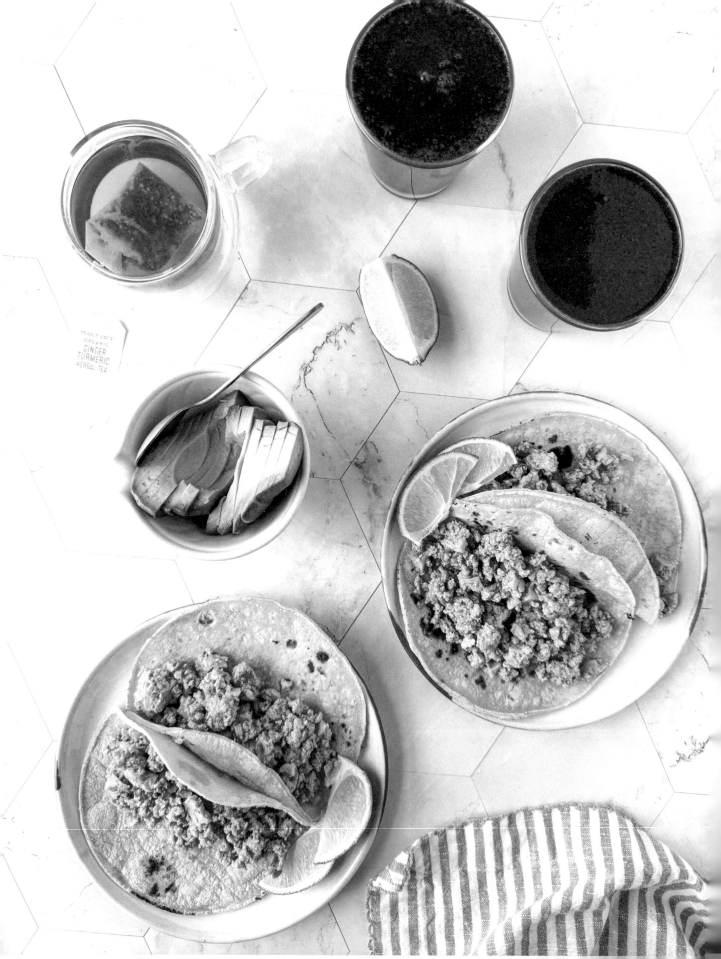

Tofu Scramble: 3 Ways

Makes about 4 servings

Crumbled tofu is sautéed and seasoned with spices, then served as a savory breakfast or main dish. The versatile base recipe offers three delicious variations—perfect for wrapping in a burrito, stuffing into a warm pita, or layering on avocado toast.

INGREDIENTS

- 1 tablespoon extra-virgin olive oil
- 1 (14 ounce) block extra-firm tofu, pressed
- ⅓ cup plain nondairy milk
- 2 tablespoons nutritional yeast
- ½ teaspoon garlic powder
- ½ teaspoon ground turmeric
- ½ teaspoon paprika
- ½ teaspoon salt

FOR SERVING, OPTIONAL

- Avocado
- Tomatoes
- Microgreens
- Toasted sourdough bread or charred tortillas

METHOD

1. To a medium bowl, crumble the tofu block into tiny pieces with your hands or a potato masher.
2. To a small bowl, whisk together the nondairy milk and dried spices.
3. Heat a large nonstick skillet over medium heat and add the oil. Once it shimmers, add the crumbled tofu and cook for 5 minutes, or until lightly golden, stirring occasionally.
4. Add the milk and spice mixture, stirring until well combined. Cook for 30 seconds to 2 minutes, until you reach desired consistency.
5. Season with salt and pepper to taste.
6. Serve on toast or tortillas with desired toppings.

VARIATIONS:

Southwest Scramble: Stir in ½ cup of your favorite salsa with the milk and spice mixture, cooking as directed. Serve in charred whole-grain tortillas topped with avocado.

Mediterranean Herb Scramble: Add 1 teaspoon dried oregano to the spices, cooking as directed. At the end, stir in ½ cup chopped fresh herbs like mint, basil, or parsley. Serve in a warmed pitas drizzled with Tzatziki Sauce (page 61).

Leftover Veggie Scramble: Reduce food waste and use up those roasted or sautéed veggies! Chop 1-2 cups of cooked veggies and toss them in the tofu, cooking as directed. Serve with avocado toast.

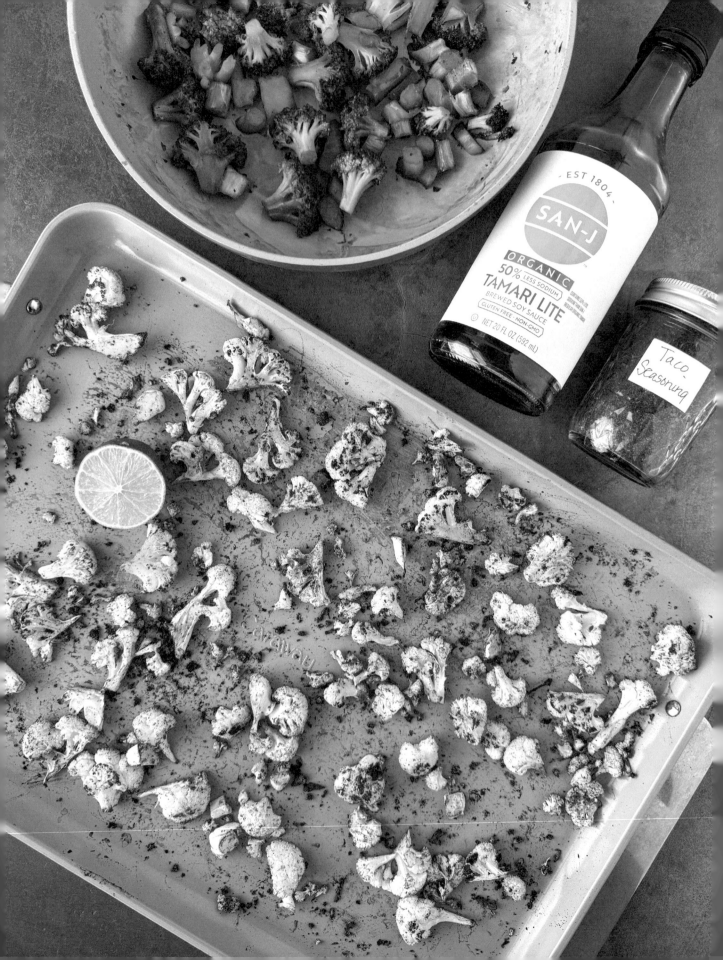

How to Cook Without Oil

Some people choose to reduce or skip oil for health reasons, and the good news is—you can still enjoy delicious, flavorful meals without it using these simple methods.

Sauté & Stir-Frying:

Cookware: Use ceramic-coated nonstick pans, enamel-coated cast iron, or heavy-bottomed stainless steel skillets for optimal results.

Use Liquid Instead of Oil: Preheat your skillet over medium heat for 1 to 2 minutes until nice and hot, then add your ingredients, stirring occasionally. Add small amounts of water or low-sodium vegetable broth as needed to prevent sticking without steaming your food.

Roasting:

Cookware: Use ceramic nonstick or stainless steel rimmed baking sheets.

Line for Easy Cleanup: Use parchment paper or a silicone mat to prevent sticking.

Boost Flavor Without Oil: Toss prepped vegetables in low-sodium tamari, citrus juice, vegetable broth, or water with your favorite spices. Spread evenly on a lined baking sheet and roast as directed.

Cooking without oil is simple, flavorful, and satisfying! With these easy swaps, you can enjoy delicious sautéed, stir-fried, and roasted meals—no oil required.

Acknowledgments

Creating this cookbook has been a journey of love, creativity, and collaboration. I am deeply grateful to everyone who has played a part in bringing it to life.

Carolyn, Kristi, Leanne, Steph, Audrey, and Gayle: Thank you for being my taste-testers, cheerleaders, and constant sources of inspiration. Your honest feedback and encouragement have shaped every recipe in this book.

Ted: This book wouldn't exist without you. Your encouragement and belief in my abilities kept me going, even when doubt crept in. From the initial concept and beautiful illustrations, you helped bring this vision to life. Thank you for being my constant support. XOX

Carolyn: Because of you, I was inspired to start my personal chef business! Thank you for your guidance and medical nutrition contributions to this cookbook—I appreciate you!

Kristi: I'm honored that you wrote the foreword and advised on this cookbook—it gave me the confidence to make it a reality. Thank you for believing in me!

Mom: My palate for real whole foods was formed by what you prepared and taught me growing up, and I am forever grateful. Even when your friends made fun of our "weird" bird food! I cherish our shared enthusiasm for farmers markets, healthy food, and recipes, always with flavor first. I love you!

Dad: Thank you for being one of my biggest cheerleaders. I know you would be so proud that I created this book. I miss you every single day, but I know you watch over me because I feel your love and warmth. Until we are together again.

Auntie Patti: To my foodie extraordinaire! Thank you for filling our kitchen with gorgeous treasures and your continued love and encouragement. I will always cherish the Pineapple Party in Paradise. Cheers, Baby Cakes!

Uncle Terry: So grateful for the unforgettable adventures over the years and the many flavors that made them even more special, such as the best homemade hummus in St. Augustine, the dragon fruit smoothie that (almost) cured our jet lag in Jakarta, and the juiciest figs from your tree in Le Peuch. Your generosity and love of good food have inspired this journey. Muah!

The book team: Thank you Kristy Twellmann for your wisdom, guidance, and detailed design of the book at a time when I needed it most. Thank you Kelly Messier for your detailed eye and thoughtful suggestions, bringing further clarity to the content and my vision.

And finally to you, the reader: Thank you for welcoming this book into your kitchen. I hope these recipes inspire you to create meals that tickle your tastebuds, nourish your body, and simplify meal prep so that you can spend more time enjoying life!

With gratitude,

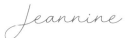

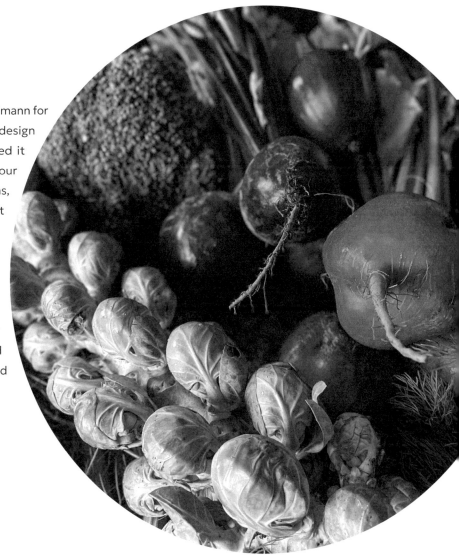

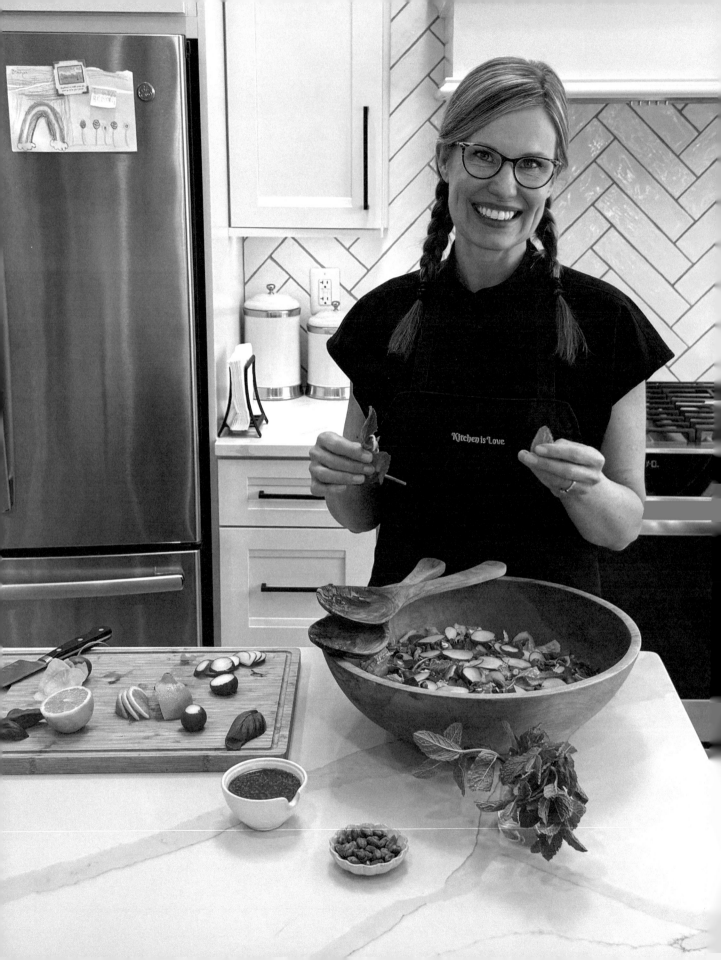

About the Author

Hi everyone! Ted here.

Let me tell you a little about Jeannine. She lifts people up. She's a patient listener, always eager to learn and honor people's traditions and challenges.

I'm especially proud of the network of lifestyle and culinary medicine practitioners she's built—friends and colleagues who share her passion for health and well-being. Jeannine has a gift for bringing their knowledge to life through flavor, texture, process, and creativity, making healthy eating approachable for all ages.

Some of her happy places include local farmers markets and being in the kitchen with her clients, helping them swap in positive habits and wholesome ingredients to crowd out the less supportive ones, one small step at a time.

Her recipes are thoughtful, reliable, and authentic. She tests them rigorously, both at home and with clients, ensuring they're as enjoyable as they are nourishing.

Jeannine wears many hats: personal chef, culinary coach, and now, first-time cookbook author. She's a certified plant-based chef and health coach, and she volunteers with Corewell Health's Culinary Medicine program and MSU Extension cooking classes. She also gives back to the community, most recently partnering with Gilda's Club to support those navigating a cancer journey.

Together, we love exploring the world—near and far—immersing ourselves in new cultures, cuisines, and communities.

She finds joy in nature, whether hiking through the forest with our dog Luna, spending time by the water, practicing yoga, kayaking, or playing pickleball.

Keep in touch with Jeannine!

Website: www.kitchenislove.com
Instagram: www.instagram.com/kitchen.is.love
Facebook: www.facebook.com/kitchenislove
LinkedIn: www.linkedin.com/in/jeannine-billups-4495831a

About the Contributor

Carolyn Vollmer, MD

Board Certified Lifestyle and Physical Medicine & Rehabilitation Physician

Dr. Vollmer is a board-certified Physical Medicine and Rehabilitation specialist who became additionally board-certified in Lifestyle Medicine. She currently works at a Lifestyle Medicine speciality practice within a large healthcare system. Due to her expertise and breadth of lifestyle medicine experience, she was recognized by the American Board of Lifestyle Medicine as a Lifestyle Medicine Intensivist in 2024. She works closely with both medical students and nationally with the American College of Lifestyle Medicine to empower patients to prevent disease and restore health through a more plant based eating pattern. She personally became whole food, plant-based after the birth of her third son and has never felt healthier. You can find her on LinkedIn to learn more.

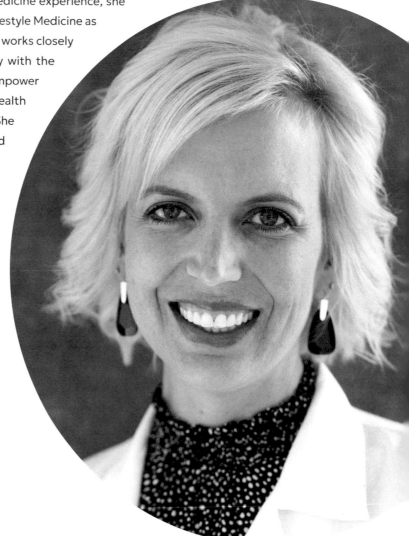

Endnotes

1. Walter Willet et al., "Food in the Anthropocene: The EAT–Lancet Commission on Healthy Diets from Sustainable Food Systems," *Lancet 393*, Issue 10170 (2019): 447–92.

2. Gary E. Fraser, Hannalore W. Bennett, Karen B. Jaceldo, and Joan Sabaté, "Effect on Body Weight of a Free 76 Kilojoule (320 Calorie) Daily Supplement of Almonds for Six Months," *Journal of the American College of Nutrition* 21, no. 3 (June 2022): 275–83.

3. Xian Wang, Zhaoping Li, Yanjun Liu, Xiaofeng Lv, and Wenying Yang, "Effects of Pistachios on Body Weight in Chinese Subjects with Metabolic Syndrome," *Nutrition Journal* 11, no. 20 (April 3, 2012).

4. Joan Sabaté, Zaida Cordero-Macintyre, Gina Siapco, Setareh Torabian, and Ella Haddad, "Does Regular Walnut Consumption Lead to Weight Gain?," British *Journal of Nutrition* 94, no. 5 (November 2005): 859–64.

5. Dagfinn Aune et al., "Nut Consumption and Risk of Cardiovascular Disease, Total Cancer, All-Cause and Cause-Specific Mortality: A Systematic Review and Dose-Response Meta-Analysis of Prospective Studies," *BMC Medicine* 15, no. 1 (December 5, 2016): 207.

Index

Z

Made in United States
Cleveland, OH
20 June 2025

17828496R00119